I0709590

Copyright © 2023 by Mary Ladd
Cover design by Kevin Barrett Kane
Internal design by Michael Zipkin

All rights reserved. No portion of this book may be reproduced without written permission from the publisher or author except as permitted by U.S. copyright law. If you would like permission to use material from this book other than for brief quotations in reviews, please contact longhaulerpub@gmail.com.

"Three Months Going on Four" first appeared in *Oxford Poetry*, Issue 94, and "Still Life with Dead Passion Fruit Vine and Dog Bowl" first appeared in *Brink*, Issue 3. Used with permission.

The content provided in this book is intended to be a source of accurate and helpful information about the subject matter and is not meant to be used or applied as a substitute for professional services or medical advice of any kind. The author and publisher do not provide professional services or medical advice and are not liable or responsible for any losses or injuries allegedly arising from any information contained in this book.

Published by Long Hauler Publishing
1663 Mission St., #602
San Francisco CA 94103

First Edition: November 2023

978-1-7356553-8-3 (Paperback IngramSpark)
978-1-7356553-9-0 (Paperback KDP Print)
979-8-9890289-0-0 (Ebook)

Cataloging-in-Publication Data is on file with the Library of Congress.

Writing and Poetry from 45 Long Haulers

THE LONG COVID READER

Edited by Mary Ladd et al.

Long Hauler Publishing

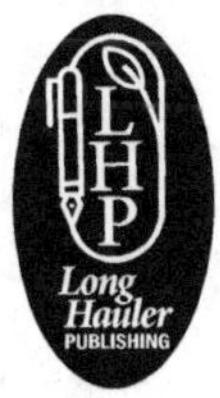

Table of Contents

INTRODUCTION

Dear Readers,

Getting the word out about the Long COVID experience is an urgent mission. Too many of us remain sick, and we can't afford to wait.

Reading this collective narrative of COVID long haulers can offer validation and connection to those wrestling with Long COVID-related symptoms. It also provides a firsthand look for friends, family, caregivers, and co-workers who seek to better understand the long haulers in their lives. Our struggles, resilience, and adaptability mirror that of tens of millions more worldwide.

Long COVID leaves us exhausted, stressed, lonely, and grieving the fuller lives we once led. Many of us are debilitated, newly disabled, or unable to participate in society anymore. It's heavy lifting to carry constantly recurring worries about new and old symptoms, waning relationships, and finding money to cover medical bills and basics, including housing and food. Fatigue, cognitive impairment, dizziness, heart palpitations, chronic cough and chest pain, post-exertional malaise, autoimmune disorders, and hundreds of other symptoms and associated conditions bring up scary questions.

How will I breathe, walk, work, sleep, eat, or show up for my loved ones?

The reality of life with Long COVID means living alongside these deferred fears, often forced to choose whether to prioritize the discomfort of today or the uncertainties of the future.

Can I afford care? Can I find answers? Can I find hope? *Can I ever recover?*

Realizing that many others faced the same symptoms, experiences, and doubts as I did felt as overwhelming as it did meaningful. By late 2022, I started thinking about *Wildfire Magazine*, a print and online publication with ongoing writing events by and for the young breast cancer community. I feel less alone reading *Wildfire*, because the text lets me feel seen and heard as a breast cancer survivor. Contributing to any writing project that connects us all has always been exciting and powerful. So, an aha moment struck: Where is the *Wildfire* for long haulers?

The Long COVID Reader features 45 contributors representing a range of ages, backgrounds, and medical experiences. I believe their stories and creative writing have the potential to challenge Long COVID preconceptions, foster understanding, and, ultimately, spur improved clinical, financial, and emotional aid programs. These curated stories, poems, and essays at once capture a spark of healing and highlight the systemic failures that have left many Long COVID patients isolated and unsupported. I hope their words can hammer home the point that anyone can experience unpredictable extended illness following a single COVID-19 infection.

This anthology is by and for the long hauler community. Bringing it to life builds on the tireless efforts already in place for post-COVID conditions, as well as the decades of momentous groundwork laid by the patient communities of ME/CFS, HIV/AIDS, chronic respiratory disease, diabetes, cancers, heart disease, autoimmune disorders, and countless others. There's no way this book would exist without the help of long hauler patient-advocates and many hardworking allies.

While it may feel more comfortable to move on from the disease, disruption, suffering, and deaths of COVID-19, those living with its effects remain desperate for greater and better support, medical care, and policy change. Amplifying the voices that have too often gone unheard — and acknowledging their extended and unwanted hardship with interest and empathy — fosters the change needed to create a more inclusive, compassionate world. Whether you're part of the Long COVID community or want to learn more, this book offers insight, understanding, and even a few giggles for levity.

We still have much to do.

Thank you for joining us,

Mary

Navigating Unfamiliar Waters

Stacy Wentworth, M.D.

FOREWORD

I was at home the day the lockdowns started. I shook our friend awake early on Saturday morning. He was visiting from France, and I urged him to get up and pack, hurrying him to the Raleigh, North Carolina, airport. We loaded his carry-on with masks, snacks, and hand sanitizer as he caught one of the last planes to Europe. Upon landing in Paris, he sent pictures of empty trains and implored us to "get all the gold and all the food." On my way home, I unenthusiastically picked up a bag of dried beans, a gallon of milk, and $100 in cash at the grocery store.

Driving to work on Monday morning, streets normally busy with commuters merging onto I-40 were eerily quiet. The medians were not yet sprinkled with discarded blue masks. At my cancer center, valets checked temperatures at the door and turned away family members required to wait in their cars. The puzzle table sat empty, and our coffee station had been cleared. A buzz of expectation hummed through the department. I returned home that first day to a makeshift decontamination area in our garage, lovingly assembled by my husband and son: Paper towels, 50/50 bleach spray, and a clothes hamper greeted me. Starting my new arrival ritual, I murmured a prayer of thanks while wiping down the inside of my car. I peeled off my scrubs and ran upstairs to wash off whatever I carried home on my body.

I ate dinner perched on the bottom of our stairs, a strategically placed mirror reflecting my son and husband at our kitchen counter. I shared the frightening COVID-19 hospitalizations posted on our intranet — a mere 10 cases at the time — and they updated me on the daily press conferences and news reports. We prepped for imminent disaster. My husband put a lock on our chicken coop and buried ammunition in our pasture. We met with a lawyer and completed our oft-delayed wills. My equine veterinarian emailed to say that his office donated personal protective equipment to my hospital and asked if we needed anything else. I wept in an empty mall parking lot, my head on the steering wheel, as love and fear overwhelmed me.

At work, radiation therapists pushed and pulled human bodies into position on the treatment tables, leaning over to see tiny tattoos hidden in folds of human flesh. "Six feet apart" was impossible. Schedules shifted as patients moved in and out of quarantine. Lonely extroverts showed up early for their appointments, supplying conversation and laughter in our socially distanced lobby. The front desk staff tirelessly explained the ever-changing visitor policy, and our nurses cajoled reluctant patients into wearing their masks properly. Furloughed administrators tried their best to lead but faded in and out of our morning huddles.

My clinic partner and I met daily, debriefing on the detailed dispatches from radiation oncology colleagues in New York and abroad. Should we shorten treatment courses to clear our machines? Would our waiting room soon be filled with critical-care beds? When would we, with just a few months of intensive care unit experience between us, be called to manage ventilators? We converted in-person consultations to phone visits, abandoning video early on as the swift transition to technology left our rural and elderly patients behind. New rules appeared in the breakroom: Don't wear watches, don't touch your face, bring your lunch from home. And new questions greeted us daily: What about our two pregnant therapists? Who should be working from home? When will we have more hand sanitizer? Gloves and masks were removed from exam rooms after frightened patients facing empty stores took supplies for themselves. I bought six full-face scuba masks on Amazon on the advice of an emergency medicine physician's post that went viral.

The steady bulwark of evidence-based practice shifted on its foundation, eroded by waves of a novel pandemic. Cancer screenings plummeted and our surgical colleagues were ultimately sent home — only the most advanced cases presented for care. For the first time in my career, the primacy of cancer treatment was questioned. Our well-defined roles shifted uncomfortably, and our once-precise departmental procedures were in constant flux. We clung to anecdotal reports, waiting anxiously to discover our own fate. Absolute certainties one week became conspiracy theories the next. Patients, now also potential disease vectors, flowed into our lives while our families were kept at bay. With their bald heads and bruised arms, the already wounded became more vulnerable. Well-crafted systems meant to protect and shield splintered around us: Our protocol-driven world of radiation oncology became an unfamiliar landscape.

Over Zoom, I asked our chaplain how to process it all. She suggested that I was surrounded by teachers; I had a front-row seat to humans surviving unexpected disruption. When I began to share, hesitantly at first, my patients graciously answered by providing me a privileged glimpse into how they coped with the uncertainty of their cancer journeys. Watching my deeply embedded boundaries be swept away by this changing tide, I now swam with them through masses of new data, strange vocabulary, and changing plans. I felt their empathy as I practiced the uninvited but necessary skill of "taking it one day at a time." As the world swirled around us, we grew closer, not just provider-to-patient but human-to-human. Cancer never stopped, and together, neither did we. It seemed that for a moment the ark was big enough to hold all of us.

Most of our patients and staff got vaccinated as soon as possible, feeling short-lived relief that at least one uncertainty had been addressed. The introduction of these miraculous vaccines, however, threw us all into strange new waters. A patient screamed in my face that I was part of a government conspiracy to inject microchips in his arm. One cancer survivor I had known for years comfortably expressed pride over his son joining an online alt-right white nationalist group: His son believed vaccines were part of a global plot to take over our country. At the feed store, empty shelves sat behind signs warning that horse dewormer was not safe for human consumption. Not accepting defeat, I handed out schedules for vaccine clinics and addressed vaccine hesitancy at every opportunity.

While patients readily accepted my recommendations to shoot invisible rays into their most precious organs, some became unhinged when I mentioned an injection with a few molecules of sugar and water. Beloved co-workers who refused mandatory vaccination were gone overnight. My responsibility as a doctor, a leader, and a trusted source of health information weighed even more heavily on every patient interaction as I plunged headlong into unfamiliar branches of medicine, learning and translating simultaneously. I joyously exhaled when patients confirmed their appointment times and felt sharp stabs of failure when others refused to engage. How could we be in the same room and yet so far apart? How could those who had trusted me with their lives now reject my pleas to grab the life-saving opportunity in front of them? When information on vaccine complications emerged, I wondered — should they?

As we move into yet another year of this pandemic, the decontamination area in my garage has long since been disassembled and I am grateful for the sanctuary of vaccines, however complex. The familiar rhythm of my clinic days has returned, and our staff has resumed their normal roles, albeit still masked. The day-to-day climate has calmed, and I don't reflexively brace when someone coughs. Questions around bodily autonomy still challenge our delicately rebuilt trust in science and medicine. Natural disasters once again uncover institutionalized inequities. I often long for the intimacy of those early months; not for the fear and certainly not the death, but for the unbounded sense of community when we were all rowing the boat together.

When I survey my internal damage, I monitor the scars from this journey. Are they healing or calcifying into a deeper fibrosis that will harden my heart? I am still broken, yet I return each day to the front lines. When I review a new patient's records and note their unvaccinated status, I only swell with sadness, not outrage. I pause as I place my hand on an exam room door with fleeting wariness, now made conscious of the possible conflict on the other side. On my best days, I take a deep breath and exhale gratitude for this one moment, this one patient, this one day.

How much healing is enough? What can be salvaged from our communal wreckage and what is lost forever? Can doctors and patients show up broken together? In the gorgeous essays that follow, COVID long haulers bear witness to this collective trauma and point us toward a future where we learn, trust, and listen. The contributors to this book, all survivors who live with Long COVID, remain largely unseen and unheard as the world pressures us to move on. In our rush, however, we have a continuing responsibility to all who survive. We must see past the acronyms or labels and reach out to these battered but unbroken souls. While these pages do not contain answers, they do hold the hope of understanding. They are a testimony that surviving this storm was enough to prompt the process of rebuilding, together. May we all rededicate ourselves to bringing better support, treatment, and quality of life to those who desperately need it.

No industry funding or other financial funding related to this project to disclose. This is an original and previously unpublished work.

Meditations in an Emergency

Andrew David King

ESSAY

Early in the pandemic, I made the mistake of browsing my conservative aunt and uncle's Facebook pages. It was a carnival of ignorance and cruelty. One meme transformed the Cat in the Hat into an anti-masker: "I will not wear one in a bar, I will not wear one in the car." A photo of a goblet glass filled with beer, a blue surgical mask wrapped around its stout middle, with the announcement that even this beer was "politically compliant." A complaint that no one can think for themselves. That humans are too unintelligent to be left to their own devices. That hopefully "Jesus will come soon." At Costco they bought 37 things, my aunt, B., says, and how many other people had touched them? And then the cashier and bagger touched them, but they couldn't hand over their membership card without wiping it off first. This proved, they thought, that it was all security theater.

One of B.'s friends posts on her timeline to say she's seen a video of someone's hand being injected with an identifier tag— "the mark of the beast," she calls it. Rather than debunk this, she replies: "Oh HELL no." And C., her husband, is a Bill Gates truther who thinks the coronavirus, or the vaccine that will serve as part of the response to it, is part of a New

World Order-type conspiracy that's about "thinning the herd," as his friend put it. One of their friends posts something as "just something to ponder": a meme that suggests the virus isn't deadly since you have to get tested to find out whether you have it.

Browsing the pages of my more liberal friends, on the other hand, you'd be forgiven for thinking the pandemic was over, or had never happened. I search for "COVID," "pandemic," and "vaccines" in my friends' past posts — hardly anything. One friend posts several times about his poem in *The New Yorker*. Another posts a recipe for tofu bites. People need to stay sane somehow, I remind myself. But is it the sane or the insane who don't talk about the tragedy in front of them? And where did that put my aunt and uncle; where did it put me?

The national news always presents footage of hospital hallways with tunnel-vision filters on them when talking about COVID statistics. Is that supposed to be the last thing a terminal COVID patient sees? Or do they see, instead, one of the gaunt, portable video conferencing stands that, in a chilling photograph that had "gone viral" on Reddit, allows the dying to speak to the images of their loved ones one final time?

The claim implicit in the news graphic seems to be that, in a hospital, you only see what's in front of you — or, worse, that hospitals present themselves in reality just as TV dramas present them, so that the dramas are no longer presenting hospitals dramatically, but merely presenting them as they are. Cases where reality apes TV — where TV, in all the derogatory senses of that term, dictates the language that fact speaks.

Georges Poulet, writing in *Studies in Human Time*, 1949: "Suffering that lasts is made up of a thousand distinct sufferings, each one of which in its own right donates its own unique and changing character to thought."

Someone I know on Facebook likes the Facebook post of someone I don't know, and that drags the post into my news feed. It's a photograph of a gathering of anti-maskers during the Spanish Flu pandemic at one of the northern entrances to Golden Gate Park, along Fulton Street.

Mask; masque; life mask; death mask (Keats', a copy of which a friend's father had hung in his library.)

The last thing my uncle posted before I unfriended him — three years into the pandemic, having moved to Austria and decided to set even firmer boundaries — was a Venn diagram with three intersecting circles. In one circle were people who believed that COVID was "real" (the word still in quotation marks, as if hedged). In another, people who believed that everyone had the "right" (my quotation marks — hedged) to wear or not wear a mask. The last included people who believed the pandemic was being used for nefarious political purposes. An arrow directed your attention to the center: "Believe it or not, it's possible to be all three."

In unfriending my aunt and uncle, was I becoming what I myself had been subjected to, what I so despised: a social ostracizer, a puritanical discourse-policer? Was I "folding"; was I calling it quits; was I giving up? More importantly, was I hindering the long-term progress I wanted to see — a saner, safer, more compassionate society?

The cases continue to pile up. I suspect that we'll soon be in worse condition than Italy. Someone on Twitter looking at the data extrapolates it two weeks into the future, following Italy, and predicts over 5,000 deaths in a single day in two weeks. Americans: "Well, the flu has still killed more people, historically." (A sudden interest in history.) And the awful rhetoric that this is "only" of concern to the elderly, the disabled, the vulnerable. Looking at circulating case studies from other countries and data about hospitalization rates, it appears that a non-negligible number of otherwise healthy young people will die horrible deaths from this — some due to the unavailability of ventilators.

Whether those will become part of the media narrative or not remains to be seen, and I'm of two minds about it: if the football star at St. Ignoramus gets sick and dies, that'll be all over the news because of the destruction of a young, attractive body — the public will want to register the damage to its delusions and nurse them back to "health." But it would be good if more young people took this seriously, saw themselves as mortal, though by the time they have even the faintest glimmer of a realization — or of their roles as vectors, which as of now it seems many are happily playing — it'll be way too late for it to have any effect.

One thinks: Here I am, reading, while they don't have enough places to put bodies in New York City. How hideous. But really, it's always been hideous, even before, when you weren't thinking about it; and, as two people in the *New York Times* comments section pointed out, one in sorrow and muted alarm and the other in desensitized matter-of-factness, it's always been the case that our economy is predicated on suffering and death. Maybe, as another says, Americans are getting what they deserve.

I associate two deaths with the lemon tree in the backyard of my father's house, neither of which are its fault.

The first is the death of Ruth Bader Ginsburg, which I learned about while on the patio, near the tree, unpacking boxes from the move back to California. I had some sense of what it meant, then, for the Supreme Court, what it would unleash upon a country already tired and assailed.

The second is a baby bird whose death, in all likelihood, I hastened by inattention. Unpacking some boxes of books stored under the awning, I'd noticed two birds who'd built a nest in the wisteria were upset — squawking, chirping, perching now on the boxes, now on the lemon tree. Pushy, I thought — defending the nest. Only half an hour later, when my dog, Clementine, reached under the tree to investigate something, did I realize that their hatchling had fallen, probably after trying to fly. I set the baby bird on the brick edge of the flower bed, but by then it was too late: it breathed a few more times and then died, a drop of blood escaping its beak.

Was there a crueler, truer parable to be told about me, I thought? To have transplanted one's awareness of the world into books, into texts, and as a result missed another's suffering. To have done so in writing. In writing this, even.

I arrive in Los Angeles from the Bay Area a few hours before my appointment with the Austrian Consulate. Their office, a sublet on Wilshire Blvd., is near the National Cemetery, so I drive there, exhausted, to pass the time and maybe take a nap. Nested between the boulevard and the freeway, it's noisy; the lawns are flat, the graves inlaid; the signage and maintenance make clear that this is not a place for the living. (An extensive list of guidelines regarding grave decorations is printed on the lid of a trash can labeled FLOWER VASES.) I look for a place to get out, to sit, but the dead have been laid away everywhere — including one person who's been stowed in the smallest possible wedge of grass between the freeway on-ramp and the cemetery's outer road. (To have died for your country, and then to be placed in economy storage ... I remember my aunt, J., pointing to the last name on the Vietnam War Memorial in D.C. and saying: "If the war had ended just a day earlier ...")

I park near one of the only benches on this side of the cemetery and get out, but the noise of the freeway is overwhelming. Then a maintenance worker comes by in a golf cart, parks, and takes out his leaf blower. I've left my earplugs at home — and here is noise. In the cemetery. Noise upon noise.

It takes me a while to understand what he's doing. He's not removing stuff, or even blowing it toward a certain area, but simply cleaning it off the headstones. Another park worker — are they part of the National Park Service, actually? — stops his riding mower, the one with an American flag pinned to it, to put some plastic flowers back in place. He seems to know by heart where they're supposed to go.

Syncope

Austin Crowley

Early this morning I am torn
awake like a scab mid-clot.
The simple thing, to stand,
is, for me, not so

simple. Feet touch the floor
already unsure. I heave
myself up and clatter
to the ground like a bundle

of wood. Blood flushes
from my head. A bottle tilted over:
right me and all the liquid
rests at the bottom.

On my back
my heart breaks me
by beating. My eyes thrum
against their sockets.

Maybe it's best I remain
down here and become dust
bunnies. They seem to live
so carefree until they're swept away.

No, I'll grow
mossy if I just lay here.
So, I press up and the world
blurs black like ink.

Never Better

Maya Lea

SHORT STORY

"Heroes Work Here!" The poster is as tall as she is and had appeared on the bare cinder-block wall of the service corridor midway through the first year of the pandemic. Its message has long since ceased to inspire. As she passes it on her way out of the building she either ignores it or, if she isn't too fried, makes up snarky variants: "Suckers Work Here!" "COVID Lives Here!" "Why Are You Still Working Here?"

The upscale retirement complex's pretentious official name is The Pinnacle. Three years after she'd caught the virus here in the early days of its first wave — by being a hero — she's still serving time at this place she's taken to calling the Plague House. Her current taglines for it are "Abode of the Entitled Old" and the less highfalutin "Home of the Snug 'n Smug." No bare cinder-block walls lit by flickering fluorescent tubes for the Golden Oldies: *they* get Tasteful Decor in *their* hallways.

Dark humor for dark times. Behind her N95, nobody can tell a grimace from a smile.

Social distancing is likewise helpful when you look like you've been to hell and haven't made it back yet. A few months into Long COVID her burning eyeballs had become perpetually rimmed in red; tiered pouches cupped by craters now hang beneath them. Under her clothes her skin is an alien landscape of volcanic eruptions and scabrous deserts. Wearing a bra hurts. Every morning before staggering out of bed she forces her throbbing legs into thick black compression hose, her bulging veins a lurid topographical map of the war waged within.

She's shrunk: hunched over and an inch and a quarter shorter. She also takes up less space sideways. Residents have been complimenting her lately on how thin she's gotten, wanting to know her secret. She should write a book and call it "The COVID Diet: Less Food, More Pills" or "Annihilate Your Appetite!" There's less and less she can eat these days as the aftereffects of COVID continue to wreak havoc on her digestive system. She's too tired to eat much anyway, dragging herself through each day on a few hours' broken sleep, wracked every night by whole-body, cell-deep pain that the doctors — even those who believe her — can't name and can't fix. But hey, lookin' goood from six feet away!

Once, maybe a year and a half ago, she'd rounded the corner in the service corridor and almost collided with a pair of residents in terry cloth bathrobes and flip-flops, each with a mask dangling jauntily from an ear, who'd apparently taken a detour en route to the spa. They were gazing up at the "Heroes Work Here!" poster. One of them had snarled, "Heroes *live* here too! What about *us*, how come *we* don't get a poster?!" Behind her mask she'd zipped her lip, refraining from pointing out that, unlike the staff, no residents had been expected to find emergency child care and sleep in this corridor night after night during lockdown. No residents had risked their lives and those of their families caring for strangers.

She'd contracted COVID in the line of duty, and the virus had taken a wrecking ball to her life. She had stepped up, done the right thing, put the welfare of "our most vulnerable" above her own — and gotten clobbered for it. So now these ingrate inmates felt they deserved their own poster for ... *what*, exactly? Because Canasta was canceled? She's exhausted, in constant pain, and facing financial ruin while they're complaining that their housekeepers are out sick, the brunch buffet isn't what it used to be, and they have to wear masks in The Lobby Shoppe.

In the spring of 2020 she had volunteered to work an extra shift, doing live-in overnight post-op care for a resident with Alzheimer's when they were short staffed and his family couldn't be bothered to come pick him up. He had just been discharged early from The Pinnacle's rehab unit, aka (Un) Skilled Nursing, because they needed his bed. At his cramped studio apartment in (Un) Assisted Living she had scrupulously followed the CDC's guidance: mask outdoors but not in, wear gloves and disinfect everything in sight.

That had been dead wrong, of course. It should have been "Don't inhale and run for your life! You have no idea what you're in for, and neither do we." The man's symptoms had begun that first nightmarish night, but it had taken her four days to get someone to pay attention. He wound up in the ICU but recovered; she wound up with Long COVID. From his posh suburb, the man's son had sent her a cheesy dime-store thank-you card with a $25 check on which he'd written "tip." Insult to injury.

Heroes worked here, paid dearly for it, and ceased to matter. As she fell into the abyss of Long COVID over the next few months, she'd had to cut her hours drastically. What she made no longer even covered her rent. She'd lost her benefits just when she needed them most, and nobody in her situation was winning disability appeals. Three years later her savings are nearly gone, eaten up by medical expenses, along with her hope. She's desperate to quit but can't afford to. She dreads setting foot in the Plague House, her PTSD ebbing and flowing in sync with the tidal rhythms of each successive variant as it sweeps through the complex.

A couple of months ago, well after the pandemic had been declared over on the 6 o'clock news, The Pinnacle had its scariest outbreak yet. The virus spread like wildfire in the wake of a Sing-Along Social in the Great Room. Soon hazmat supply carts parked outside apartments dotted the tastefully decorated hallways, the modern equivalent of red Xs on plague victims' doors. Surreally, life continued much as usual for those Golden Oldies who hadn't (yet) tested positive. Snug 'n smug in the belief that *they* couldn't catch COVID, few of them put their masks back on or canceled their dinner plans, even as more and more of their neighbors fell ill, even when one of the hospitalized residents succumbed.

The Pinnacle's president, aware of the inverse correlation between case counts and occupancy rates, doubled down on his Potemkin village approach to damage control. He was ably abetted in this institutional ass-covering by the incompetence of his Head of (Un) Health, aka Commander COVID, who clearly couldn't run a testing program to save his life — or anybody else's. She's long since given up trying to find the missing supplies or suggest solutions. These days she just goes through the motions like the rest of them. The shambolic testing program's bogus case counts keep everyone happy: investors, residents, the public health department, and the marketing team.

At the end of the service corridor she pushes open a heavy metal door and steps outside, tearing off her N95 to gulp fresh air. Commander COVID huddles behind the shrubbery at the edge of the parking lot, sneaking a smoke — unmasked in more ways than one. She hesitates, wondering whether she's supposed to pretend she hasn't spotted him. She decides it's too late for that, so she waves. He waves back, calling, "Long time no see." Only for the entire past three years, she thinks. "How ya doin'?" he asks.

"Never better!" she replies, knowing he won't get it, "So long." She heads for the exit.

Third Illeversary, March 2023

Pato Hebert

ESSAY

Today is my illeversary. I stumble into year four of living with the virus' reservoirs of resolve, COVID-19's toll on the body and spirit. A sore throat was my first warning sign on March 2, 2020. A symptom so subtle yet common that the emerging medical guidance assured it was no sign at all. They didn't know I'd inhaled a floating ember of the wildfire infection. Tissue as tinder. The issue is tender. Swiped out.

Four days ago, a raging soreness once again enveloped my throat. It seemed to come out of nowhere, except chronic illness is everywhere. In the body. Our collective body. This fragile, magnificent body opens up with a throat. Sick. Scratch. Scrape. Shout. Sore. Sour.

I have stubbornly insisted on a long-hauling existence that is far more than just dour. Whenever I speak on patient panels, organizing roundtables, advocacy briefings, or kiki sessions, and somebody asks what I want other folks living with Long COVID to know, I usually make candid mention of the relentless struggle that requires great pacing, patience, diligence, mutual aid, interconnectedness, and care. And then I emphasize celebration and vitality. The fierce richness with which our disabled lives can thrive. The sacred power of breathing and being, together.

There is also the harrowing sorrow of no tomorrows for all who have died. Even as federal, state, and local governments declare an end to our emergency, those of us living with loss and Long COVID know the dangers of such narrow-minded decrees. With its markups and takedowns, the market will not save us. Our resolve just might.

Tonight and every day, a need to remember, recalibrate, replenish, reinvigorate, reconfigure, and renew. I want to insist on an existence of vitality and rest, imagination and joy. It helps, even if it does not always go so well. I begin year four masked around others and unmasked in my exhaustion. Massive sleep disruptions persist despite constant tinkering and revised attempts to medicate, meditate, and despair a way toward rest. Brain fog, disorganization, lost thoughts, and missing words conspire against my wishes and will.

COVID-19 impacts so many bodily systems. My lungs occasionally still struggle for a full inhale, though the pool has helped restore some confidence and rhythm. Ghost pains jab, ripple, and taunt across my torso despite the successful surgery in December 2021. My thermostat lives only in extremes. Cold will stay stuck in muscles, tendons, and bones. Sweat will begin to pour at the slightest provocation — exertion, anxiety, frustration, desire, fear. It can take an hour for the glands to glance at the clock and decide it's time for a break. Sheets still soak. Throat still rasps. Temples and frontal lobe throb.

The most painful ongoing symptom set in for good last summer: a completely fried nervous system. My mood board is like a secondhand shop where the wonderful games aisle has been knocked upside down with pieces strewed about. Third eye in search of a new prescription. Even if I somatically scan to find, feel and release the tension, it floods right back minutes later without me even realizing it. I end up in yet another flex that wrecks any possibility of supple ease or flow. My thighs, in particular, seem constantly tense and sore. Regular swims have strengthened these quads so they now can carry me up stairs or spring hillsides that my lungs can now almost navigate without gasps. But it feels like my nerves are fraying from the inside out. Surrounding tissue all swole. Swell.

One of my most common symptoms is constant crying due to the pseudobulbar affect. I have been trying to write a piece about all the different forms this crying takes. Weeps. Drips. Gushes. Pours. Floods. Moans. Mists. Hydrates. Helps. Hiccups. Sobs. Squeals. Spasms. Flows. Appreciates. Signals. Releases. Frees. A precipitation index amid so much drought.

I have a smidgen more awareness now, a few helpful tricks, oodles of compxs, queridxs, and a loving crip community. I need them all when the ache or wail or regurge bubbles up from the depths. Four years in, I still have insurance, not because it's a right but because I labor against my health and because although Long COVID is a designated disability, disability benefits are almost impossible for long haulers to secure. Structural insecurity. So, many systems of inequity have been exacerbated by this putrid pandemic.

It's just after 3 a.m. here in New York. The recent snows have mostly melted, and the streets are quiet on my walk home save for some cars crawling along the thoroughfare and distinctly repeated "Fuck yous" caroming off buildings from a distance. It's just after midnight back home in Los Angeles, and the relentless rains of the climate crisis have slowed again. It's just about time for me to make something, anything. If I were at an artist residency that came with an endoscopy camera, I'd deep throat the probe and screen grab what it sees. Instead, I try to swallow my phone to reach the screaming and keep on dreaming — the paradox of screen as care.

Today is also my daddy's birthday. I've already sent him a bouquet of various yellow flowers. But I will reach out to him later, after lying down and seeing what this body wants and needs, will allow for or resist. The last time I saw him was Nov. 2 as he and my mother and sister exited my small apartment. They'd barely settled in for a rare stay, but they had to leave because I'd tested positive for reinfection, and we wanted to keep them safe. Five months without hugging him, eight months since any extended quality time. But he is still alive, and so am I, and this is a special song worth singing.

Toxic Positivity

Rachel Robles

ESSAY

A few months ago, I was talking with an acquaintance, updating them on my life and progress, when they asked, "So what else is going on besides all that sickness stuff?" It was heartbreaking because this person meant well. By steering the conversation away from my illness, they intended to focus on the other parts of my life, the more "positive" aspects. However, the flaw in that approach is that illness seeps into every part of a chronically ill person's life, whether they like it or not. With the advent of this question, my options to share became limited. I could not share how proud I was for reading a book because that would have reminded them that, at one point, I was too sick to read. I could not share how I can now endure an entire workday without crashing. Suddenly, my whole life had become too "negative," causing discomfort to those without a similar experience.

This isolating experience is typical. I have felt the discomfort of silence many times after mentioning a small aspect of my life, such as a doctor's appointment, to a group of people. In that silence, I hear them say, "Why is she *OK* with this life?" and "She's supposed to say '... but I'm going to get better!' and not burden us with this." While that may not necessarily be what they think, that's what they say in their silence.

For some reason, people need to tell you to "think positively" when you're sick. I'm not sure how all chronically ill people react to this statement, but the phrase immediately makes me recoil. It's not the content of the message that makes me recoil. Creating hope, acknowledging gratitude, and conveying empathy are all powerful practices that support any person's physical, emotional, and mental well-being. No, it's not that. It's the context in which this phrase is used. Much like how the term "all lives matter" invalidates those harmed by systemic racism, "think positively" has been used to silence the legitimate experiences, fears, grief, and callous injustices happening to chronically ill and/or disabled people.

I just want the right to talk about my lived experience, free of stigma. I want to talk about the mundane, like how much I enjoy watching the clouds go by my window when I'm resting on the couch. I want to talk about my fascination with the nervous system and phytonutrients. I want to talk about my anxiety about keeping up with an able-bodied world. And I want to talk about the systems in place that keep my fellow spoonies and me from navigating our disabled lives successfully.

While people think wiping away all hints of negativity helps, their likely well-intentioned efforts turn our lived experiences into a taboo, where our feelings and realities are edited out. That's neater and tidier than reality. Making illness too taboo to mention and discuss may seem helpful, since it removes even a hint of the uncomfortable and negative. Yet this process also fully ignores and erases every aspect — positive, negative, and everything in between — of a chronically ill person's life. Our days and experiences have many "in-between" moments. It's time we face, acknowledge, and process them.

From My Hospital Bed

Steven Lewis

"... for when I am weak, then I am strong." St. Paul (2 Cor 12:1-10)

So I've wandered this far into the breath-
taking woods, nothing but darkness ahead,
nothing behind except what I think

I remember. Or perhaps made up. I don't
know. Also, I don't know how I know
but I know now there is no path out

of this infinite forest nor why I am
certain there is a fallen tree trunk
up ahead that I will come upon and

sit down, lean over and, pressing my bare
forearms onto my weary thighs, gaze out
through the inscrutable thicket: branches,

leaves, choking vines, waiting for whatever
comes next: animal, rain, morning, hunger,
faith, love, the hunger of love, the everything

and nothing that arrives when prayers
are but childhood wishes, when we know
in our scarred and perfect souls

that what is sacred is profane, profane
sacred, that there is merciful strength
in closing our eyes and welcoming

this illness
of being human
with an unknowing smile.

Ode to this Frail Body

Steven Lewis

For Leigh and Isabel who wondered

So you find yourself
lying in a hospital bed
on your back, needles
in your arm, cannula
up your nose, intermittent
pneumatic compression
devices on your legs,
and you're staring up
into the darkness, when
some 3 a.m. voice arrives
like a drunk call, or maybe
like some nightshift orderly,
a former professional athlete
in gown and gloves who
empties the waste basket
and says behind a mask,

If you make it through
the night, there will be
no standing ovation
awaiting you in the morning.
There are no fourth quarter
Hail Marys that make any
difference in this life, silly man,
no prizes, no film contracts,
no eureka, no aha, nothing
ahead but the flesh and some
daily practice, something you
do every day as sustenance,
as a reminder among other
daily reminders like hunger,
that you do not exist at the behest
of who you think you are passing
through this life, you are here
at the merciful mercy of the frail
and tender body in which you live,
in which you have always lived,
as you were in the beginning
and as you will be at the end.

And in that moment of darkness,
you see that no matter what
you've done between your first

yowling breath and this dark night,
there has been no sanctum outside
the body, that even if you rise
from the bed, shed the hospital gown,
and dance wildly in the moonlight
to the pulsing light on the monitor,
passing ghosts in the hallway,
and enter the world beyond
which only blasphemers dare
describe, there is still only this
sickly body to render you alive.

So you take a shallow breath and wait
patiently for morning, where your daily
practice awaits you, some sweet devotion
without purpose beyond itself, beyond
superstition, even beyond hope, leading
you closer and closer to some fleeting
reconciliation for the day you are alive,
some breath of labor or art or prayer
that begins to fade the instant you breathe
into it, even as it burrows by rote under
your skin, pulses through your arteries,
the in and out of your aching lungs.

I Had This Amazing Life

Amy S.

ESSAY

For just about 25 years, I worked for nonprofit organizations that provided services for domestic violence and human trafficking victims and survivors and worked toward social change with regard to gender-based violence. For almost 20 of those years, I worked at the executive level, and many considered me to be an advocate, mentor, and leader, dedicated to guiding people and processes for the better. The work was fast-paced and emotionally and mentally challenging, but I was inspired almost every day by the staff and the survivors and that fueled me through the many hard days.

This was more than a job; it was a career, which was and remains a massive part of my identity. So, who would I be now that Long COVID left me unable to work and advocate for others?

About a year into Long COVID, I felt fortunate to find an excellent therapist who has ME/CFS, known as Chronic Fatigue Syndrome. She has slowly helped me grieve the life I once knew and work toward accepting my current limitations. I learned from her about Dr. Gabor Maté's work. Maté teaches about how stress and trauma contribute to disease, addiction, and chronic illness. In his book *When the Body Says No: Exploring the Stress-Disease Connection,* he urges the reader to ask essential questions rather than masking emotions with positive thinking; questions such as "What is not in balance? What have I ignored? What is my body saying no to?" In one of his talks, he reads aloud obituaries of people who died from various diseases, noting that the things that were touted as their accomplishments or passions are the same things that killed them — for example, being lauded for loving their job so much that they worked right through their chemotherapy treatments, only stopping a few days before their death. Maté states that this compulsive need to identify so closely with the work that one does rather than the physical and emotional needs of the self is a big risk factor for illness.

While I spent the first half of my Long COVID illness questioning how this disease could have happened to *me* — a 44-year-old frequent exerciser, hiker, and volleyball player who for decades ate a vegetarian/pescatarian diet — Maté's work led me to understand that this same — healthy — person was also someone who was almost always running on fumes professionally, most days of the week, for decades. My hours were long and intense, jam-packed with meeting after meeting — talking, thinking, and decision-making — often followed by managing the inevitable evening or weekend crises involved in helping adults and children at risk of serious harm or even death at the hands of their abusers or traffickers.

For two-and-a-half years, I tried so hard to push through and keep working either full-time or part-time, when the reality was that my health was worsening. How could it not? It was a lot for a healthy person to manage, let alone one with crippling fatigue and other debilitating symptoms. At some point, I knew what I was risking if I kept up the pace — bed confinement, perhaps for the rest of my life. It was time to loosen my grip and let go of the delusion that I was still in control.

About three months into my second Long COVID medical leave in two years, I realized I had to surrender since I was not recovering at all. I wrote this "look back" journal entry in the past tense soon after as a way to process how I would feel in the future, having given up such a vital part of my existence:

August 2022

I had this amazing life. I had a career that was borne out of passion, that scared some and awed others. I was smart, kind, humble, outspoken, introspective, forgiving, generous. I changed some lives for the better. It all changed me for the better. I taught and was taught, in an endless loop.

It was hard, maybe the hardest thing I've ever done. It pushed me to my very limit. It forced me to feel a vast range of emotions, the most intense emotions that could be felt. It broke my heart, even while making me manically happy.

It made me more raw and tired than I ever could have imagined. It betrayed me and then begged forgiveness, over and over, a "honeymoon" cycle of sorts. It frayed my nerves to shreds as it simultaneously numbed and strengthened me. It rewarded me for my loyalty and long hours by letting an evil, opportunistic virus into my body, threatening my livelihood. It almost led to my demise. And still, I kept giving it everything I had to give ... until I had nothing left.

I hate what it's done to me. I love what it's made me. It was the fullest career I could have had, marked by the ups and downs of learning, failing, and succeeding in helping others. Yet I know I cannot return to it. This illness sparked a deep awakening in my conscience, for which I am grateful: giving all of myself to a career to the extent that it poses risks to my health and possibly to my life is something I no longer have to accept. I can care passionately about a cause and still stop short of total self-sacrifice.

This Vase Won't Hold Water Anymore

Vanessa Svihla

ESSAY

At first, I measured time in days. Five days of Paxlovid. Ten days in a hotel room far from home. Eight days until I could leave my hotel room with a mask. This disease, along with the Centers for Disease Control and Prevention (CDC), my physician, and antigen tests held agency over me. It was frustrating and scary but simple and straightforward. I easily held on to silver linings: I wasn't getting anyone else sick and was fortunate that the prolonged hotel stay would not be a financial burden.

Days shifted to weeks, punctuated with tests and measurements — a chest X-ray, vials and vials worth of blood work, a transthoracic echocardiogram with bubble study — to assess a laundry list of lingering symptoms: chest pain, anosmia (loss of smell), weight loss, fatigue, tachycardia (fast heart rate), brain fog, headaches, dizziness, strained vocal cords, memory issues, poor sleep. And more silver linings: my lungs, heart, and blood were healthy. These test results held agency over my trust in my experience. Was I unknowingly malingering?

But my symptoms rang out like a bell, louder than self-doubt. The fatigue grew stronger than me — like a late afternoon, impossibly long shadow overtaking my previously high-energy self.

Another bit of fortune: Medical professionals believed me. My chart reads "COVID-19 long hauler." Yet most medical professionals offered little more than cold comfort: "It's just so new. We don't know anything yet." The absence of guidelines mitigated their agency, shaping what they were willing to try: tests, not treatments.

Suddenly, boldly, my physician took a host of actions. I took a short course of prednisone, but there was no change. There was also a test for postural orthostatic tachycardia syndrome (POTS), a condition in which patients get dizzy or faint upon standing; their heart rate typically increases by more than 30 beats per minute. It is an autonomic nervous system disorder — a type of dysautonomia. My physician said my test results were not quite normal — finally, evidence validating that something was wrong. She gave me a printed sheaf of papers I would come to know as the "CHOP," named for the Children's Hospital of Philadelphia, which created this much-circulated protocol.

This protocol, originally developed by Dr. Benjamin D. Levine, is a research-backed exercise program for treating POTS. The original version was provided only to doctors, but eventually, the Children's Hospital of Philadelphia produced a version for patients. This version includes instructions for calculating heart rates, guidance on strength training, and eight months of training schedules that begin with recumbent exercise and gradually scale into intensive, daily upright exercise like jogging. (We'll come back to the CHOP.)

As I wept in her office, my physician offered and I declined mirtazapine for my mood, which she consistently described as "appropriate." She also wrote a referral for occupational therapy. The young occupational therapist was suspicious of post-exertional malaise, and he encouraged me to "push harder." Post-exertional malaise is well-documented among long haulers; it is when physical and/or mental exertion produces fatigue one to three days after the exertion. Experts concur that pushing harder is not advisable. He also suggested using a rollator which could make me "feel less nervous." I purchased one, not to "feel less nervous" but because having a wheeled mobility device, with handlebars and a built-in seat, allowed me to avoid fainting while standing.

My physician wrote a heart monitor referral, which I declined because that modern, wearable stick-on device was contraindicated by my allergic contact dermatitis. She offered a referral for physical therapy, which I declined initially — feeling overwhelmed by appointments where I was *somebody else's problem*. And then she left, joining a faraway practice. I believe her boldness came from knowing she was leaving.

Weeks became months. I navigated work, setting shorter meetings that gave me time to lie down. I discovered more silver linings: When my student tells me about their chronic illness, empathy is easy; I finally learned to say "No" to work opportunities and service overloads.

I started the CHOP. A friend with a clear POTS diagnosis invited me to a social media group for people like us. Again, I was fortunate: I had a lap pool where I could swim, which is the only CHOP-approved form of recumbent exercise that my hypermobile joints could withstand. I missed a couple of sessions and struggled with progress, intimidated and judged by the eight months of exercises on pages scattered across my table and floor. I was lucky to have had so much experience with Excel, which made it comparatively easy (though time-consuming) to turn the rigid CHOP into a living, dynamic tool that made it palatable to repeat weeks and shift schedules as needed. Some dragons were waiting in month four because the training modes were limited to exercises I knew I could not do.

When I contacted my doctor's office, they submitted the PT referral my physician had offered. Initially, they paired me with a PT whose expertise was the vestibular system "for dizziness." I was again *somebody else's problem*. Weeks later, I finally found someone willing to test and treat at the consult with the new PT. I shared resources and details; she contacted a colleague with POTS. Together, we adapted, improvised, and strategized. Even with her support, months four and five of CHOP were difficult. There were six to seven hours of exercise most weeks, and I knew that each upcoming cardio would be more challenging each time. A phrase haunted me throughout the months of CHOP: "Striving, never arriving."

As I write this, I am starting month six of CHOP. My symptoms are much improved, yet that trendline is hard to notice. I live in the noise of experience, always at the edges of my capacity, always striving. I feel like a knocked-over vase that has been haphazardly glued back together and placed *just so*. From certain angles, from a distance, everything seems OK. On closer inspection, you realize *this vase won't hold water anymore*. That does not mean it cannot serve a similar purpose. This vase can hold dried flowers, just as it is.

Dried flowers remind us of what was — a ghost of their vibrant past, lacking their former perfume, an appropriately anosmic experience. And when these reminders are troublesome or unpleasant, perhaps the vase will be pushed to a dark spot in the cupboard, where it is easier to forget. I sometimes experience this when I try to reconnect with colleagues in new, less convenient ways. It is hard not to apologize for being broken. But with careful effort, we can bring the broken pieces together again, edge them with gold and the toxic sap of the urushi (or lacquer) tree, making a new object that celebrates its scars. Unapologetic.

When I shared this broken vase metaphor with a colleague, it was one of the first times I disclosed Long COVID's impact to someone outside my immediate circle. It was oddly reassuring that he missed the seriousness and related it to something like a sprained ankle, offering advice about toughing it out. Another silver lining: If no one cares enough to notice, I might just get away with being this broken vase for as long as it takes to do that careful remaking.

With all these silver linings, I must surely be fully electroplated by now. Even so, I feel stalked by the next infection and the undoing it may bring.

The Illness That Keeps on Giving

Ellen Belluomini MacKenzie

ESSAY

Pre-pandemic life seems surreal to me now. Two years before COVID-19 hit, I started the job of my dreams developing a new master's in social work program. My blog and academic writing were garnering attention. My part-time work as a consultant, training various organizations and academic programs on integrating technology into social work education and practice, was prospering. The future of social work was becoming a hot topic in academic circles, and I was receiving invitations to speak from around the country. Little did I know the significant turn my life, along with everyone else's, would take as COVID-19 became a global pandemic.

I contracted COVID-19 twice, first in early March 2020 and again that June. My partner's career as an essential worker increased our risk. Truthfully, she didn't believe the seriousness of COVID-19. Her precautions were haphazard, and she brought COVID-19 home. Twice. With the first infection, she developed a high fever and I had tightness in my chest. We slept almost nonstop for three days. We each lost the sense of taste and smell, but our symptoms abated rather quickly. Our cases were never confirmed though, as, at the time, only hospitalized people were being tested for the virus.

Then came another bout three months later. Contracting COVID-19 a second time increased our initial symptoms from the first exposure. Her fever rose to 104.3, and the ER sent her home, the doctor instructing her to come back if it reached 105.1. "Doesn't brain damage start at 104.5?" I asked myself, worried for her health. When her fever broke, she began to recover but had little memory of her time with a fever. Then I became ill, but I thought it couldn't be COVID-19 because I had no congestion or breathing difficulties. But when the tightness and pain in my chest increased, I went to the hospital.

At the Johns Hopkins Emergency Room, I was immediately taken back to a room. Sheets of opaque plastic lined the walls and machines, giving the look of a construction site rather than an ER. Lying on my hospital cot, I attended work meetings by Zoom and waited for my test results. My work came to an abrupt stop when a nurse came in to tell me I was having a heart attack.

I waited in fear for hours as tests were ordered and reordered. Behind the curtain to my right, a man had OD'd on a drug. I listened as the team brought him back to life five times. Each time I waited with bated breath, hoping he would live. The ER team succeeded; he lived. To my left, a gentleman coughed until I thought his lungs would come out. I hurt just listening to the phlegm work its way out of his chest. After a childhood riddled with bronchitis, I feared contracting COVID-19. A heart attack seemed a better alternative to COVID-19 — anything seemed preferable to not being able to breathe.

After a 12-hour wait in the Emergency Room, I was admitted to the COVID-19 floor.

"Why am I on the COVID-19 floor? I tested negative in the waiting room," I asked. The doctor, through a screen on an iPad, stated, "We usually need to administer two to three tests before people test positive for COVID-19."

The new room terrified me. People in full Centers for Disease Control and Prevention body gear came out of a tent-like structure that blocked the doorway to my room. A loud machine with tubes piped to the outside clamored away. Nurses entered my room, dressed in outfits that looked like they were pulled from the set of a movie that is a cross between an apocalypse and *Twenty Thousand Leagues Under the Sea*.

Twenty-four hours later, the cardiac team informed me that my test results indicated a COVID-19 infection, explaining that some COVID-19 patients experience heart-related symptoms, rather than respiratory issues. They needed my room for sicker patients. I was discharged and went home to recover with instructions to follow up with a cardiologist.

Weeks, then months, passed, and my symptoms didn't decrease. At 56, I had never taken heart medication. Now I had a cardiologist and high blood pressure. My mind could not focus on work. Fatigue became my nemesis. I napped for two to three hours, three or four times a day, and then I would sleep the entire night. But fatigue was not the only symptom. I remember throwing away an expensive hot sauce infused with truffles because "this must be a bad batch. I can't taste the truffles at all." I questioned my sanity along with my health.

A college professor's work schedule is flexible. A 9-to-5 job would have been impossible to navigate, and disability would have been my only option. But grading student papers became a significant struggle. I would grade a few assignments, then need to rest. Despite being a prolific reader,

I could no longer follow complex storylines. Even audiobooks were not an option. My creativity evaporated with the illness. I would forget about tasks or appointments at work.

I researched my symptoms, knowing something was not right with my body. I found a Facebook group dedicated to people experiencing Long COVID (now medically called Post-Acute Sequelae of SARS-CoV-2 or PASC). The Facebook group validated my symptoms and shared current research findings. Most importantly, I didn't feel alone and crazy anymore.

Complications from Long COVID continued. My partner brought home pink eye a few months after our second infection. Her symptoms lasted three days. For me, it was a different story. I had such severe swelling that I could not fully close either eye. The inflammation led to three weeks of blindness. I could not open my eyes without the feeling of a thousand needles piercing them. All day and most nights, the pain kept me up. Specialists could not relieve the symptoms or help the agony. Due to the restriction of drugs during the opioid crisis, pain medication was not an option. I visited eye specialists for nine months. The damage to my right eye is permanent. My vision changed from -4.25 to -7.25, and I now struggle with dry eyes, impaired night vision, and fluctuating visual acuity.

In addition to the fatigue and brain fog, I experienced many other symptoms, including exhaustion after working out, dizziness from standing up, a strange rhythm to my heart, and unusual sweating. One night, I got up to use the bathroom. I never made it. My dizziness was so intense that I blacked out in the bathroom. When I fell, my face hit the corner of the door, then the ceramic tile. My partner found me on the floor, bleeding. My two front teeth had cracked off, and I sustained a broken nose. In the aftermath, my life consisted of working, sleeping, dental reconstruction, and more visits with specialists.

A year and a half after my initial COVID-19 infection, blood tests indicated I had a high level of anti-nuclear antibodies (ANA). The National Institutes of Health identify ANA as a defining feature of autoimmune connective tissue disease. My positive ANA test resulted in a rheumatoid arthritis (RA) diagnosis. I continued my research, which led me to a hypothesis and subsequent studies indicating that my SARS-CoV-2 infection triggered an autoimmune response that led to the development of RA. All my Long COVID symptoms blended with this new diagnosis. Questions plagued me. Do I still have Long COVID? Will my RA be permanent? Is this illness the "new" me? How do I get back to being functional again? What will people think if I can't be a high performer at my university? Will I lose my career?

I still don't have answers to all these questions, but a year of trying different drug regimens led me to a medication that has addressed most of my symptoms. I am not symptom-free, but I am not getting worse. And I have learned to manage my illness. I schedule time to recuperate if I travel or participate in activities with friends or family. Working out requires time to rest. My old motto, "Work hard, play hard," is a remnant of the past. I have experienced each stage of grief over my lost health: denial, anger, depression, and bargaining, and I move closer to acceptance every day.

COVID-19 has changed my entire life, but I have grown along with the losses. I am learning about work-life balance, and my quality of life is improving. No longer a workhorse, I value my downtime. I ask for help more often. I practice meditation and mindfulness to expand my peacefulness.

Creativity has become the barometer of my self-care. If I am mindful of my energy, my mind allows me to be creative in art. My artist's life is blossoming. Better late than never, I am enjoying the work-life balance I should have learned 30 years ago. Through this illness, I am finally home to myself.

Still Breathing

Shell St. James

I lie motionless on threadbare sheets, suspiciously watching the ceiling.

The cracks in the white plaster change every day, like a mirror, mocking the lines on my face.

Am I awake? Maybe I'm asleep.

Maybe I'm dying, but don't know it yet.

Maybe you are, too.

We dream out loud, over endless cups of coffee, of escaping the confines of this prison.

We dream of sunshine.

We dream of rain.

The smell of the ocean. The taste of snowflakes.

I try astral projection in secret, pretending to listen to music, my headphones muted. I want nothing more than to leave behind this room, this body, this existence.

Go somewhere green, somewhere healthy. Somewhere happy.

I fail, remaining tethered to the pale woman on the sagging green couch.

The ceiling fan casts shadows on my body, slicing it into sections. The dark stripes erase half of my form, but you stare at the TV, unaware that I'm fading away.

I wait, as instructed. The words echo in my mind: "wait and see."

It's a pointless thing to say. I've wasted so much time—perhaps half of my life—waiting.

Waiting for green lights, for daylight.

For darkness, for weekends.

You switch off the TV, and the silence hurts my ears.

I study you from beneath my lashes. You've become the only person in my entire world, but our forced proximity reveals what strangers we really are.

I withdraw further, shrinking into myself, hiding in my flannel robe.

You hide behind your sunglasses.

There is no sun.

The planet continues to spin, apathetic. The human race is inconsequential.

Mankind teeters, six feet apart and clinging to memories. We tumble through the day, the month, the year. Solitary and numb.

There's a 2022 calendar hanging in the kitchen. It puzzles me. Time itself seems off-kilter.

I rip off the bottom half, leaving only the pictures. The days of the week have lost all identity. Rounding them up, we christen them only: today, tomorrow, and someday.

It's been two years. "Someday" has arrived for most of the world.

But you and I are stuck in this loop.

Still breathing, but not living.

A revolving door of doctors offer platitudes, saying, Give it time. You'll be better soon. Back to your old self.

I don't think I can be that person again.

I don't even remember who she was.

And Breathe

Ann Wallace

ESSAY

I was upstairs in my bedroom struggling to get dressed when the delivery man arrived. My 16-year-old daughter tentatively answered the door of our long-quarantined house to the man in the vestibule, who was masked and at a distance. He placed the equipment down and backed away. "I'm not allowed to come in," he told Molly as he explained how to operate the oxygen concentrator.

When I made my way carefully down the stairs, I saw that Molly had plugged the bulky black concentrator into an outlet in the kitchen. She had attached the longest stretch of green tubing, 50 feet, that the man had left, giving me just enough range to walk upstairs at night for bed. More than a month into my illness — one that would extend well beyond two years and involve more than 90 symptoms impacting nearly every organ system in my body — my lifeline had finally arrived. In our naiveté, we had expected a tank like scuba divers wear, one that would empty and need to be refilled. But this machine pulled air in and fed it back to me in a condensed form. Molly turned it on with the flip of a switch. I hooked the tubing around my ears and placed the nasal cannula under my nose. The rhythmic whoosh began, soon becoming the background pulse of the house.

Molly, my younger daughter Abby, and I laughed as I took a few selfies, exhausted but almost giddy with the relief of oxygen pumping into my body. Securing supplemental oxygen had been no small feat: Normally, it has to be authorized by a visiting nurse who measures the patients' oxygen saturation, but no nurse was going to come to the home of a COVID-positive patient now. After I nearly blacked out during a rare in-person appointment, my doctor, clad head-to-toe in PPE, was visibly concerned. She jotted down my oxygen levels and tasked a case worker with securing the equipment for me. The concentrator arrived, along with a tall emergency tank and a smaller portable one in a backpack, a few days later.

It was April 2020, and for five weeks every day had been filled with the terror of my unsteady oxygen, my near blackouts when I stood or even spoke. As bad as the days were, the nights were worse. I had not slept for more than three or four hours at a time in weeks. Each night, I woke after a few short hours of fitful sleep, my head throbbing and legs vibrating with pain from hypoxia. I would lie curled in a ball, clutching the base of my aching skull and rocking back and forth through the darkest hours. And each night, as I quietly begged for the pain to stop, I listened to Molly — infected with COVID a week before me — coughing, coughing, coughing in her room. Every night on end, the same tortured routine as I waited for the sun to rise.

I know now that I never should have been home alone, riding this virus out with my daughters. But hospitals were full that spring, and, truthfully, they seemed like a place where COVID patients went to die. Two of my friends already had.

The arrival of my supplemental oxygen brought a new hope and, potentially, a new way through this virus. Together we named the tank Ruth Bader Ginsburg, a summoning of her indomitable spirit to carry me through the next four weeks when the concentrator was running 24/7. Even as I began weaning myself off round-the-clock oxygen a month later, walking indoors for two minutes, then three, then eventually a walk down the block and back, I still relied upon RBG to steady my oxygen levels after exertion or to help me through my daily afternoon crash. More than a year later, I still needed it from time to time. And, worse, Molly did too, as her own Long COVID symptoms increased. When she became short of breath, she knew to put the oxygen on and stabilize her breathing.

Twenty months post-infection, Molly was away at college and still struggling, but I graduated from my COVID rehab program. I began running, not far and not fast, but actually running. I was not fully recovered and still had serious symptoms that would persist for another year or more, but I no longer needed supplemental oxygen. That fall, I placed the concentrator and my emergency tank in my vestibule and went inside to sign on to a Zoom call. While I was occupied with my meeting, a delivery man came and picked up RBG, the removal as silent and contactless as the delivery so many months earlier. My front hallway, where the equipment had lived these many months, felt empty.

In the days that followed, whenever I noticed pressure in my chest or my breath grew short, I felt a small and momentary panic that I was on my own again. I kept a supply of tubing and cannulas and full masks, most of them mine but some labeled with Molly's name, even after RBG was taken away. I felt safer having those remnants of the machine that just may have been responsible for keeping me alive.

As I was tidying up a couple of months later, I saw the tubes and masks sitting on a shelf. I gathered them up and held them in my hands for a minute. Then I walked to the kitchen trash bin and threw them all away.

My COVID Journey

Sabrina McQueen Johnson

The mental and emotional stress of Long COVID has been hard for me and my family. Before my COVID-19 diagnosis, I led a fully active life that included family, work, and friends. I was a professional educator, serving over 26 years as a teacher, education specialist, and principal. I've been married for 25 years and have a teenage son. I love to read, dance, travel, and spend time with my family and friends. However, since November 2020, most of these activities have been limited or nonexistent for physical and mental health reasons.

ESSAY

I spent over two months in the hospital fighting COVID-19 and was released from a rehabilitation center in January 2021. My mind and emotions had become fragile because of the lack of information about COVID-19. There was still a great deal of confusion about treatment and the long-term care of patients like me with extended hospital stays. While in the hospital, I could not have any visitors, which took a toll on my mental health. I'm family-oriented, so this was hard, especially because I was sick. I had so many doctors, nurses, and specialists coming in and out of my room that I could not mentally keep up with everything they told me. When I would speak to my husband or siblings at night, I struggled to remember everything that happened each day.

Days got long, and the nights were even longer. I continued to rely on my faith and prayer, as others prayed for me. There were days I felt mentally defeated and struggled to breathe. However, I could not give up. When my mother-in-law passed away on New Year's Eve from COVID-19, the walls of isolation closed in even more. She died just two weeks after the death of three colleagues. I was frustrated, tormented, and mentally exhausted by the thought that I could not be there to emotionally support my husband and son.

After the hospital discharge, I was still not mentally prepared for the pain of grief to absorb my thoughts and hold me mentally hostage. Just as I laid in the hospital bed for two months, I sat in the same place on the couch for almost two years. I was still afraid of COVID-19, as other variants were coming out. I did not want to leave the house or socialize with anybody outside of my immediate family. I limited my television programming because too many COVID-19 stories were on the news.

COVID-19 left me oxygen-dependent, another reason I did not want to go anywhere. I had to use silver oxygen tanks for almost a year, and I did not like that they would run out and need to be changed so often. Even with my new portable oxygen, I would still become short of breath with regular activities. Home health care nurses, therapists, and my family encouraged me to breathe and move around. I was glued to the sofa and my pain.

My friend, a mental health nurse practitioner, suggested I talk to someone professionally to address my mental health. I did not resist; I could not even process what was wrong. After a while, I understood what she was talking about. She scheduled an appointment with a telehealth therapist until I was strong enough to make an in-person visit. My grief was so hard that I could not understand. I was hurt, angry, depressed, and lost. I was experiencing rapid heart rates along with the other thousand diagnoses COVID-19 left me with: pulmonary fibrosis, congestive heart failure, severe acid reflux, nodules on vocal cords, COVID-19 rash, etc. I continued to rely on my faith and pray as others prayed for me.

I just wanted things to be like they were before COVID-19. I just wanted to be better. I just wanted my mother-in-law back. Emotionally, I was hurt, disappointed, and angry. COVID-19 had robbed me of so many things that I wasn't just angry; I was livid. Then there were the days I was simply numb. I could not talk about COVID-19 or feel anything because I was shocked by how my life and the world around me had changed. My COVID-19 experience was now different from those who did not have a diagnosis or those who did not get sick.

I was diagnosed with adjustment disorder, depression, and anxiety. I finally had to retire from my job as a principal at the point I thought I was getting better with my emotions. However, I became even more depressed and did not understand why. My therapist explained to me I was grieving my job and retirement. It was another loss. I did not think about my retirement like that, but it made sense. My teachers and staff were like my work family, and I love my students as if they were my own children. I loved what I did as a principal, which made the retirement transition hard. Once again, my days got long and my nights even longer.

For the first year of my COVID-19 diagnosis, I held on to the fact that I would return to work. Then, when I retired, I had nothing to look forward to. I couldn't think about doing anything I said I wanted to do once I retired because I was on oxygen and unable to do it. I'm not able to travel like I want to or start a new career or adventure. I was very sad and lonely. The phone calls and visits had begun to slow down. Everybody was at work, and I was home alone. Going to my pulmonary rehab visits was the highlight of my week.

Writing a book about my Long COVID experience allowed me to share my testimony about surviving COVID-19 with prayer. I had always written things for people but I couldn't even write a page for this book. Even when I would write a few pages, I had to quit. When I talked to my therapist, I explained what I thought was writer's block, but it was really the trauma I experienced with my COVID-19 diagnosis. Sharing those events was painful to write and read because I harbored so much anger, hurt, and pain from both the physical and mental scars of COVID-19.

I was bitter with others and myself for getting diagnosed with Long COVID. I was constantly on an emotional roller coaster. Things that were once so simple to me had become challenging. I would have anxiety about decisions for my child. I did not want to leave the house or go anywhere with anyone other than my husband or siblings. Eventually, my anxiety settled down and I would ride with others, but it was only during the day. I had major anxiety about being out of the house at night. However, I could readjust to a more active life with therapy and support from my family and friends. My therapist suggested I start driving small distances to regain some of my independence. I'm now driving only short distances, outside of heavy traffic hours.

I had days where I would just sit and stare for hours. I did not know this was a part of my depression, which paralyzed me for many days. I remember the day I released it all. I wanted to go and visit our extended families, whom I had not seen in almost three years. On the day we were preparing to visit my husband's hometown, my anxiety was very high. I told my husband I needed to lie down or cancel the trip. I was nervous, shaking, and had a headache. After I woke up from a nap, I had a big, ugly cry for no reason. I told my husband I was ready to go when my cry ended. I realized I was still grieving my mother-in-law because I did not attend her funeral service.

The prospect of going to my husband's hometown brought on all of those heavy emotions. Once I cried, I felt better. Since that day, however, I have become more active; I empower myself with my faith, family, and friends to support my recovery journey. As a Long COVID survivor, I now serve as a patient advocate and help others who live with Long COVID.

Heartsink

Emily Fraser

They call us the *heartsink patients*
because we don't get better
but we don't die either.
We just keep coming back,
making them lose confidence
until they can't take it anymore—
and then they refer us to Psych.

This Body

Emily Fraser

This body, skin of pale
crepe paper, veins blue
and snaking, rivers sloshing
with saltwater sludge.

This body, brain gritty, stuffed
with sand-swept cotton,
a Carolina beach highway
straight through the skull.

This body, weighted by
sickness, held upright by
fury. Heart, a rusty red bicycle
peddling feverish, uphill.

This body, caged tiger,
desired, discarded. So still,
so quiet—slight swish
of the tail.

This body, vessel of ancient
knowing, map of movement
through mountains, ancestors
who suffered, survived.

This body, soft creature,
permeable membrane,
imperfect, impermanent,
improbable home.

A Perfect Day in a Broken Body

Emily Fraser

First, forget perfect. Forget day.
Forget body. Forget everything. Just
breathe. One at a time. Each breath
a secret triumph. Imagine them
as pearls on a string. Watch them
add up. Flick them from left to right
with an invisible tongue. Notice the sun
streaming through the window. Feel
its warmth on your skin. Drink water.
Wiggle your toes. The heart's erratic beats?
Thank them for striving. Don't dwell
on the body as burden. Feel grateful
that it's cared for at all. Marvel
that it's carried you this far. Don't think
of MRI machines, collapsing veins,
the wind tunnel inside your head. Don't
entertain the urge to crawl out of your skin,
leaving the body behind like a cicada's shell.
Just breathe. One at a time. Here come
Nick's footsteps, shaking the floor.
Brace yourself against the vibration.

Know he brings kindness. A cup of tea.

A slice of orange. Say thank you.

Say I love you. Let it be enough.

Exile

Emily Fraser

The body I grew up with—was just beginning to grow fond of—began to speak. Quietly at first—but insistently—she whispered, *Please slow down.* I ignored her of course, but my body kept speaking. *Slow down please. I need you to slow down.* I told my husband what my body was saying. He said, *you probably just need a weekend away.* I told my doctor what my body was saying. She said, *your lab work looks great!* I told my friends what my body was saying. They said, *I think it's just our mid-thirties.* I told my body, *you'll be fine, keep going.* I even told her, *I'll buy you a massage.*

My body roared in a voice that deafened, an earthquake vibrating out from her core. The long *O* of *NO*, resounding like thunder—an ultimatum—a lamentation—a curse. I asked my body, *are you okay?—body?* But she didn't hear me, didn't listen, didn't care. Eyes spitting embers, she leaned in and hissed, *It's time to settle the score.*

Collateral Damage

Emily Pinkerton

ESSAY

I caught COVID in March 2020, despite sheltering in place for two weeks before the Bay Area rolled out its official stay-at-home mandates. From that first evening, I started live-tweeting and posting my symptoms on Instagram stories. I did it because I was terrified. I lived far from my family. My roommates took the shelter-in-place mandates as suggestions, *even after I was symptomatic*. The most my friends could do was bring groceries to my doorstep while I waved from a nearby balcony, wearing an N95 mask and standing 6 to 20 feet away, for good measure. I hoped having a personal connection to COVID would convince people to take safety measures seriously. For a while, it worked.

My guiding philosophy was simple: *there is a horrible death plague going around, I have been unfortunate enough to catch it, and the least y'all motherfuckers can do is bear witness to what I am struggling with.* This kept me connected to people who cared, who were also scared, who wanted to know how I was doing. But when I didn't get better, it stopped working. After a few weeks, people were tired of hearing me talking about my symptoms. I wasn't better, but they didn't want to know. There were visible signs of irritation (and, of course, a few subtweets) when I mentioned things like continued caution being necessary for people who were immunocompromised or still

ill, like me. People wanted to just go on their summer road trips in peace. I was killing the vibe.

Before I got sick, just as the pandemic was ramping up in the U.S., I was thinking about my mom. It was the end of February, close to the last date I saw her alive. The seventh anniversary of her death would follow a few weeks later. I was thinking about the long weeks and months where my mother lived in an incredibly difficult state: blind from tumors, unable to consume food except through a feeding tube implanted into her stomach, hallucinating and in pain. Despite all that, she still wanted to live, and said so explicitly. I thought about what I would do in the same situation. *There's no way I'd make it,* I thought. *I'm not that tough.*

COVID taught me that my line of thinking was ableism in its purest internalized form, the idea of mind over matter, mind over the body, ideas of bodies and immune systems as things we can always control, instead of precarious houses of cards. Everything in my body hurt to extremes and there was nothing I could do about it: my lungs felt like they had several small cactuses in them and were also being stretched thin so the cactus spikes would permeate deeper with each breath. The spaces beneath each joint hurt as though I were a nonagenarian who'd had severe arthritis my whole life — absolutely blistering aches. My brainstem felt like it was on fire. My breathing was labored, difficult, and painful. My heart was overworked, pounding. I never had enough oxygen. According to current criteria, my oxygen saturation crashing to 87 as I lay at rest meant I should have been hospitalized — but in March 2020, the advice I received from the harried nurse on the triage line was "Don't go to the hospital unless your lips turn blue or you lose control of your bowels," so I stayed home.

My acute infection lasted for three weeks. In the months after that, I worked painstakingly to rehabilitate my body and brain, and was met with comments like "I's so crazy how some people just don't get better!" or "Still sick, huh?" when I described, I thought triumphantly, all the things that I was now able to do (Walk a block! Write an email! Stand long enough to make dinner!) as a result of my efforts. It sounded like my value was tied to a binary: sick or healthy. One clearly mattered more than the other, and according to friends who had never had COVID, the transit between the two was quick, like walking through a doorway. I felt more that I was journeying through a vast expanse between these two spaces, an autonomous zone between places with fuzzy, poorly demarcated borders. No one seemed able to see that journey except for me and others who lived with chronic illness.

People don't mean to be harmful; they mean for you to have an easier time. Most people don't want to hold space for pain — yours, their own, anyone else's. To acknowledge that their beliefs often create — rather than resolve — pain for people like you, is too much for them to bear. They wish to sweep you into their system, to resolve your pain, so they might not have to look at it and feel pain or discomfort themselves.

This was clear to me when my mom died. Everyone wanted to ask how I was doing. No one wanted to know the real answer to that question. They only wanted to express their concern. They wanted to help right up until the moment where helping would involve feeling any fraction of pain.

The same sentiment flared when I met up with one of the roommates who'd flouted the stay-at-home mandate. She talked about the reading series she ran then and runs now — how they'd returned to doing indoor events at a dive bar we both love. She mentioned other organizers who were more strict about enforcing protective rules, with a slightly guilty, wistful note in her voice. I told her I understood. I did not say that I understood because every time I asked for basic accommodations for my health and safety as a now-immunocompromised person, I was treated as an overly neurotic buzzkill. People assume that what is fine for them will be fine for everyone.

Imagine if you could go back to March 2020 and tell yourself, "Yeah, we have a similar case rate to what we did then, and 20 percent of the people who get it have disabling long-term symptoms, but most people just pretend like it's not a big deal anymore and catch it two to six times a year." Remember how scared we were in March 2020, the bodies piled in refrigerated trucks, pop-up hospitals in parking lots, the mass graves. Imagine telling your March 2020 self that now we've decided it's OK, actually, because now more people get disabled or die from complications *months after* their infection instead of *during* the infection's acute stage. It's OK that teenagers are being diagnosed with dementia and going septic after infection number two. It's fine! We can eat indoors now! There are at least three undiagnosed COVID cases for every positive test we count now. It's fine!

When I spoke to my friend, I wanted to tell her how, for six months after my initial infection, I couldn't write or do research for my manuscript, one of the most important and meaningful things in my life — because my language and reasoning skills were too impaired to form complex ideas, much less complex sentences. I wanted to tell her how I'd get dizzy spells if I talked for more than a few minutes at once or sang too much, how my vision would frequently black out and I'd go woozy just from standing up; how I'd learned to grab furniture because I knew I was close to fainting. I wondered if she'd noticed how I got aphasia mid-sentence as we talked. Instead, I watched her bristle at the mere mention of the steps I have to take to care for myself, and I knew she was extremely uncomfortable with knowing about the limitations or difficult work of my recovery. I saw the same fretful withdrawal I had seen after my mom died; the flinching at an honest response, because merely *hearing* about what I was going through was too hard for them. They just wanted me to know they cared, hoped that could be enough, as if their words had any corresponding action behind them.

When people see me now, they want to see the weekend bike ride I am occasionally able to do. They want to see the joyful laughter that follows. They don't see that I ride at approximately six miles per hour now (extremely slow), with many stops, and a heart rate that still comes in around 150 (abnormally high for such a slow pace). They don't want to see the days earlier in the same week where I woke up in crushing pain, unable to stop my heart from pounding even as I sat around doing nothing. They don't want to see me lie down for an hour after a simple walk around my neighborhood because it was that draining. My oxygen saturation now crashes into the low 80s (sometimes even the 70s) when I simply stand or walk around my house, something usually only seen in older people with COPD (they're advised to go to the hospital at 84 percent, but my doctors assure me I don't need to worry that my readings are below this threshold). People want me to have what they have, and I don't. I have ongoing symptoms and the knowledge that my death and disability are worth it for them to have a fun night out. It's fine.

Keep Pressing On

Mary Jo Mettler

ESSAY

In spring 2020, when most community businesses and all churches were told to cease operations until the State of Alaska said otherwise, I respected my employer's orders to work from home. I sheltered in place, but, as a single person, I opted to form a "quaranteam" with another family. We beat the odds until mid-November 2020. First, one of us tested positive. Then all but one of the rest of us did.

My acute Covid-19 symptoms were mild to moderate, and I managed my care at home and made a telehealth appointment with a nurse practitioner. I already used a daily asthma inhaler, but she prescribed vitamins, supplements, and two kinds of nebulizer medications, and told me to lie prone for a specified length of time each day. I was required to test negative twice before being permitted to return to work and eventually did so.

Thinking I was in the clear and expecting my lingering symptoms to resolve any day, I returned to my job as a licensed professional counselor when my mandatory isolation period ended. But everything was twice as challenging for me as before getting Covid-19, especially administrative and computer tasks. Also concerning was my inability to make it up a short flight of stairs without stopping several times to lean against the wall, regain my balance and catch my breath while my heart rate had time to slow. The lightheadedness was frightening, and I began to worry that I'd fall each time I used the stairs at my office.

It wasn't until Dec. 9, about a month after my infection, that my co-worker witnessed one of my episodes at a store — where I was standing on flat ground — while we were shopping for program supplies together. I initially resisted her strong encouragement to seek medical attention but eventually went to the nearby urgent care facility. They immediately referred me to the hospital due to its better testing capabilities. In the emergency department, when all my test results were normal, the doctor asked me if I thought the chest pain I complained of was due to anxiety. I told him what I thought of that assumption and went home, disappointed at the lack of answers.

The following afternoon, the emergency room physician called me. There was urgency in his voice as he explained that the CT scan of my chest had been re-reviewed by another provider. I had pneumonia. He was calling a prescription into my pharmacy, and he was emphatic that I pick it up and begin taking it immediately. I complied with his instructions.

My pneumonia slowly improved, but I continued to experience a multitude of symptoms that affected my entire body: intense brain fog and confusion, short-term memory loss, inability to find words or construct sentences, intermittent stuttering, inability to concentrate, headaches, tingling in my fingertips and toes, burning sensations on my arms and other areas of my body, shortness of breath, ringing in my ears, increased sensory overload, lightheadedness, loss of balance that worsened toward the end of each day, and life-altering fatigue. My sense of smell was sporadically altered, so food might sometimes taste like pure salt or my toothpaste like wet dog. My oxygen saturation levels were often low, and my heart rate would jump from 58 beats per minute to 132 just from standing, turning over in bed or other ordinary movements. Sometimes it happened while I was sitting still.

One week after the emergency room visit, I was trying to write something on a piece of paper. I could not physically or mentally generate the words I needed. A friend was standing nearby, and I was doing my best to shield my incompetence from her, stifling my frustration and terror. But when she walked over to talk to me, she looked down at my page and saw that I'd scribbled a jagged line that trailed off and away from the few words I'd managed to write. I covered my face with both hands and burst into tears.

My head ached, and as the day wore on, the pain worsened exponentially. My speech began to slur when I spoke and I had increased difficulty finding words. My friend urged me to return to the hospital. After receiving tests, IV medication, and fluids, the doctor and her nurse explained that I was likely experiencing Long COVID. The nurse expressed compassion and concern, and shared that her sibling was experiencing many of the same symptoms. The doctor was sympathetic as she explained that the medical community didn't know much yet about Long COVID, its prognosis, or its treatment. Knowing that any acute medical concerns had been ruled out, I made my way to my car and headed home to recuperate before beginning another workday as my sole provider.

Over the past two and a half years, I've worked with my primary care doctor and tried countless treatments: homeopathy, vitamins and supplements, occasional short-term steroids, acupuncture, functional medicine, deep tissue and craniosacral massage, myofascial release, neurofeedback, cold laser treatments, counseling (EMDR, sensorimotor psychotherapy, havening techniques, cognitive-behavioral therapy, EFT tapping, and more), sound healing, external vagal nerve stimulation using the Pulsetto device, and infrared sauna. I've recently found relief from stellate ganglion and celiac plexus blocks, as well as ketamine treatments. These have helped reduce my pain, including joint pain and the sensation of my skin burning, and improved my stamina, breathing, and heart rate.

I've seen a dietitian to maximize nutritional benefits and reduce inflammation, and a cardiologist and an internal medicine doctor to strengthen my lungs and heart. I've done breathing exercises with an Airofit device, walked for rehabilitation and done restorative yoga, and my next goal is weight training. I'd like to try hyperbaric oxygen, but it's not readily available in my area.

One internal medicine physician told me that it's not uncommon for Long COVID patients to have symptoms or qualify for a diagnosis of postural orthostatic tachycardia syndrome (POTS) and/or myalgic encephalomyelitis/chronic fatigue syndrome (ME/CFS). But rather than doing formal testing for POTS, she advised me to respect my "energy envelope" and to make lifestyle changes appropriate for those diagnosed with POTS.

Socially and mentally, Long COVID (now formally known as Post-Acute Sequelae of COVID, or PASC) has been a rough ride for me. Each day contains a grab bag of unpredictable symptoms that range in severity. I have sporadic flare-ups, which can spark days or weeks of increased symptoms. I feel frustrated by my inability to plan and commit to meeting with friends in the evenings or on weekends due to fatigue. It has caused damage to relationships I hold dear. It is frustrating and sad for me to notice the difference between my pre-COVID baseline and what I can do right now. I feel like my own body is gaslighting me because the effects of PASC are real, yet most of my test results are normal. I had a fragile nervous system before having COVID, and it is becoming known that the virus targets and exacerbates the body's preexisting weaknesses.

I have navigated deep valleys and lived through some very dark days, weeks, and, at times, months with this long illness. It has required persistence and a willingness to step outside of my comfort zone in many ways. Long COVID has stripped me of my ability to mask my struggles. I've had to rely on the support system God's so graciously blessed me with to keep moving forward in my growth and healing, no matter how slowly.

As bestselling author David Perlmutter, M.D., reminds his followers, "Strive for progress, not perfection." Forward is forward, even if I move only an inch at a time. I have to make a conscious effort not to fall into "all or nothing" thinking and to be patient with myself. I'm learning to respect my energy envelope while at the same time figuring out what I am capable of doing — and making myself do it. I'm also learning the value of discovering, focusing on and savoring things that bring me joy, like singing in a trio at church (it was all I could do to find enough breath to make it through a song at first), watching my African dwarf frogs, enjoying quality time with loved ones, snuggling with animals, swinging in a hammock, watching the Kenai River roll by, or closing my eyes in the sun and breathing the crisp Alaskan air.

To my fellow long haulers, hang in there. You are believed, valued, and not alone. Together we will adapt and overcome. Keep pressing on.

We the People: A Long COVID Constitution

Anastasia Jill

ESSAY

Death shall crawl into your bones and make himself a home. Here, he will stay put and refuse to leave. You will carry him everywhere; feed, wash, and clothe him carefully in cotton. You are his mother, and he, your new son, is a parasite. Why wouldn't he be? Your body has given him no reason to leave.

Vested in your sickness, he will find the vigor necessary to wreak havoc on a system that stays so sick. Each breath will be thick with tar, and your heart will be a chunk of concrete hanging heavy in your chest where he will nurse until he's weaned. There will be nothing left of you when you're cured.

If. If you're cured —

Don't count on it.

II.

He shall have the power to impose and excise wellness as he sees fit:

hair will fall in willow-soft waves, and your teeth will rot at the root;
blanch skin will shrivel, hanging off sore brown bones;
brain will sit in your skull like a wrinkled old man sitting on the porch

swing of your jaw, idyllic and simple and empty, and without a unique thought ever again;

lungs will become useless, unloved jelly beans, each saccharine breath held down with the weight of an endless cough;

nose will not smell, and tongue will not taste;

legs will not walk, and arms will not lift;

kidneys may swell and fail with thirst carved itself into your throat, the body engorged with fatigue and waste;

bones and muscle and sinew and nerve will collapse into a mass grave of chronic fatigue; and,

This will be normal.

Your new normal.

Will you ever be well?

Probably not.

III.

The body shall make no efforts to tame the beast unleashed within. It is illegal to fight a virus some say doesn't exist.

Meanwhile, he will attack your soul and leave an inflamed, angry warrior. Upon the vagus nerve will his sword hack until there is nothing left. Because he is tired, war-torn, and traumatized. And this shall be traumatic for you; fighting his war and losing.

The fatigue is crushing. He will be a metal jaw that unearths pain you never knew you could feel. You shall have no strength to nourish your body, let alone heal, and you will fester under flesh that once seemed so ripe.

Have you ever seen a rotten heart? You will, after the war. You will develop illnesses doctors have never seen. So enmeshed with illness, you will be a battleground, a memorial to a young healthy life. Your ribs will be abandoned trenches, bullets pockmarking your back. Still, ask around —

Some will say, "What war? That never happened, OK?"

IV.

Your bowels will be on fire. No one wants to hear this, but it's true. It will not be cute, proper, or ladylike, but it's true. Your organs will turn to excrement, and your nerves succumb to the flame. Sputum will make a rainbow of mucus in oranges, browns, and greens. Your urine will be opaque and warm like a cloudy diamond emerging from the blazing coals. It is worthless, dehydrating. You will have night sweats and body odor. This is on the outside.

The inside is much worse. Any mental health conditions shall be exacerbated, a sponge for the pathogens that incite and instigate. You shall be angry and anxious and depressed and manic. You will want to die but fear such a disgustingly close reality.

V.

You shall do all the right things: take supplements, eat salads, and go on walks. You shall take elderberries and magnesium capsules. Thick spoonfuls of turmeric and ginger will coat your throat. Pills the size of your thumb will lodge themselves in your scarred, purple tonsils, be absorbed into the bloodstream, then do nothing. You shall snort sunshine and shove yoga mats directly up your ass.

You shall eat the superfoods and do the physical therapy. You will inject yourself with vitamins. Clean needles won't just break the skin but rip it like paper. You will bleed and bleed and bleed, and then you will bruise, your body adopting a mottled hue. You shall, somehow, eat too much or not enough and move the same. You will be sore and world-worn and still be told —

"Maybe you're just depressed."

You shall take stupid suggestions from those who've never been sick. You shall field unsolicited questions about your mental health. And when that deteriorates, too, you will tell them, "That's not it. I'm trying, I am. I'm not getting better, but I am trying."

They will say, "Not hard enough."

VI.

Above all else, you will be angry. You shall nurse this anger like a newborn babe. The same fetus draining your life is the one you will feed, more than even yourself. The parasite-son returns, or never really left. The rage that fuels you is also your undoing, your demise.

No one else shall wear a mask; yours is surgically attached to your face.

No one else shall keep their distance; you walk with them lashed onto your back.

No one else shall acknowledge the dying once you become one of them, least of all you.

Their ignorance shall daily be the trocar that digs lesions in your armor. Soon, you will have no protection, or you never really had any. You shall be doomed to sickness every day, forever and again. No one will come to help you.

They will only cough in your face.

VII.

You will not survive the virus twice. Most days, you won't care anymore: Let the sickness come. What are you saving yourself for? Society is going back to normal. Few distance, fewer mask, even fewer vaccinate. And above all else, is blame —

"You're sick because you're fat."

"You're sick because you're old."

"You're sick because you were already disabled."

"It's just a virus. We'll all get it eventually."

It's not eugenics. "Only the strong survive," until they're the patient anesthetized upon the table. But for now, it's just you. You are the one who is sick. You are a human person who still deserves healing, respect, but —

You shall dig your own grave with your own feeble hands. This dirt will be more nutrient-rich than you and you will be blamed for the sinkholes in your tomb. You will tend to wounds; endless, pinkish maws that threaten to consume all of your skin. You will be blamed for allowing them to stay exposed for so long. And you will find a future, a new one with accommodations, and then be called lazy for not doing what you could before. You will be fine, eventually. But eventually ain't on any calendar you can buy. Months will pass, and you will still be sick. Eventually cannot come soon enough. It may never come at all.

Suddenly, you are part of we: A community of those now mold-green around the gills and being forced to swim with great white sharks. We, who were once and remain sick. We —

We the People

have rights, just like you.

We the People

are still ill, when no one is listening.

We the People

express ourselves, while we still can speak.

We the People

ordain ourselves again, to take up the space from which we've been erased.

We the People

the sick and frail;

the disabled;

the newly, chronically ill;

We the People

do declare this: We deserve to live.

I Wish They Knew

Lisa Carpentier

ESSAY

I cry so easily. It takes very little to trigger the thin veil to break and bring the tears out. I was so strong before all of this. My body is weak, in pain, confused, clumsy, and fatigued. I was the one people came to for help, and now I can't even help myself. My mind and emotions spiral down so low I can't see a way back up. I don't have anything left of myself. I miss me. I miss working. I never knew anything but working and taking care of my family. My identity has been ripped away from me.

I didn't want to lose everything. I didn't want to lose myself. I worked hard to get to where I was, and now it's all gone. How can anyone think it's as simple as just getting up and going on like nothing is wrong? How can anyone think I haven't tried to push through this? My pride caused me to try to go back to normal, and my body fought me so hard that I couldn't win. I fought the doctors, returned to work, and tried to be my old self. It backfired. I ended up worse. Now I am disabled. I don't wish this on anyone, but sometimes I wish they could experience this for a single day to understand this fight …

I wish they knew this doesn't just give survivors a lingering cough or a little fatigue.

Some of us lost everything we had worked for.

Once independent, we now rely on others.

We are confused and frustrated, unable to remember things or complete a thought.

The pain and numbness some of us feel in our bodies isn't just something we can simply "shake off."

Depression is new to some of us, and we don't know how to feel normal again.

We suffer the humiliation of losing our jobs because we can't remember how or what to do and can't physically perform the labor anymore.

We wish they knew what it's like not to have any answers.

We wish they knew the anxiety over bill collectors calling because we already emptied our savings.

We wish they knew that this isn't something we can resolve by telling ourselves to "suck it up and deal with it."

We wish they knew the fear we feel every time our heart rates skyrocket and a feeling of faintness pulls us down to the floor.

We are exhausted all day but unable to sleep at night.

We have no control over our bodies anymore.

We wish they knew the shame of being so weak.

We wish they knew the disappointment when hopes for normalcy again are crushed.

We wish they knew this is our new normal.

We wish they knew the guilt we feel that we survived, and, simultaneously, died.

We wish they knew how afraid we are of tomorrow.

I wish they knew what we know.

A Time for PASCUA

Nelson White

"... a light sedative keeps you comfortable."

SHORT STORY

PROGRAM UPLOADING

I wake to the scent of freshly tilled earth. I am in a fetal position with my head down, arms holding my knees against my chest. All is dark. In the silence, my heartbeat comes to me. I hear its steady rhythm, thankful for some reason I don't understand. I am detached; no memory, no recognition of self. I sleep.

UPLOAD COMPLETE. INTERFACE COMPLETE.

I wake again to the same nothingness. What was once soothing is now tiresome. My mind reaches out for something, anything. Am I still asleep?

COMMAND EXECUTED. IMAGERY EVOKED.

A memory flashes, recalling a trip to Japan to see the cherry blossoms. A song dances in my mind, "sa-ku-ra, sa-ku-ra ..." I remember the crisp spring air. A cherry tree appears, a sapling only a few feet tall, its spindly branches bare.

TWO-WAY COMMUNICATION STABLE.

"Brilliant! It's working."

I imagine a canopy of cherry trees now, their far-reaching branches filling my vision. Their leaves rustle softly. They line in a row, flanking the moat, just as I'd seen at the Imperial Palace. They shelter my sapling from wind and rain. Soft, springy grass blankets the ground. I bask in the sun as it warms me, making me drowsy. Soporific, that's the word. Lovely. I roll the word around, feeling its effect. I sleep.

"Amazing what the mind can build. I named the program PASCUA, Latin for Easter or Passover, for resurrection or passage."

INITIATING PHASE II.

I wake and look for my sapling. Oh, but it's grown! A young tree with glossy green leaves, its roots stretch beyond me, reaching for water.

I follow them to the surrounding rows. The moat comes into view.

The wind picks up, generating wavelets as it travels across the moat. I lose myself in its peaceful rhythm. Water slaps the side of the stone walls, startling me. I'm in a memory, a photograph I'd taken of this very scene. Confused, I retreat.

ERROR. SIGNAL ATTENUATED. CHECK LEAD WIRE.

Everything vanishes. I fall into darkness, into silence.

"No worries, love, a minor setback. Off to radiology. Get OR on standby."

INITIATING PHASE II.

I wake. My tree is fully grown. It has a sturdy trunk, knobby gray bark, and thick, deep roots. Its branches reach wide, overhanging the moat. One leaf remains green now. The others have yellowed, capitulating to the season. The wind sidles around me. I shiver. How long have I been here? Sounds reach me: kids laughing, dry leaves crunching, a baby babbling nonsense. A low voice rumbles. It's familiar, though I can't grasp why. I dismiss it, even as a remnant trails me into sleep.

COMMAND EXECUTED.

"... entering the longest phase, a hibernation of sorts, like a winter. It's a period of deep sleep, awakening in spring."

My ears fill with the drip-drip-dripping of snowmelt falling from above. The sun is distant and pale. My tree is budding: fuzzy, white-tipped beads cover the branches. I spy a Japanese warbler on a branch with a twig in its beak; a harbinger of spring. Another joins the first. They're building a nest, choosing my tree for their home. I whisper to my tree, "Hold tight, life is precious."

TWO-WAY COMMUNICATION STABLE.

"We've moved past the halfway point. This is the resurrection phase."

Wind rushes through the trees, swirling cherry blossoms around me, filling the sweet air. I inhale deeply. Pale pink wisps land gently on the ground. Others float on the water, adding to a delicate petal-strewn blanket. The warbler flies to her nest, offering food to her chicks. All this from one sapling, *my* sapling. This was *my* creation. I built this world, nurtured it, bringing it the sun and water. And yet, despite its splendor, I am bereft. Alone, I can share this with no one. Blessed sleep takes me again.

ANALYZING DATA.

"Hold on, love. Almost there."

I look for my tree. The flowers are gone, replaced by little red berries from a bright ruby-red to the darkest burgundy. My warblers flit from one bunch of berries to another. I've journeyed through all the seasons. Is this all there is?

UNCOUPLING PROGRAM. FADING BACKGROUND.

"Mr. Hart, are you ready?"

I hear a singsong murmuring. I concentrate and the deep, rumbly voice comes into focus.

" . . . lived happily ever after."

"Read the dragon part again."

"I love this story."

I know these voices: my children, my husband. I drag myself from my pastoral world.

"You're awake!" My children scramble into my hospital bed. With her cherubic face, Posy snuggles up against me, hugging my waist with one arm while clutching a storybook tightly in the other. I hold her close. West snuggles in on my other side, taking my hand in his, his serious frown melting away. He pops his thumb in his mouth, yawning around it before closing his eyes. Colin rises to greet me from a narrow hospital recliner, an uncertain smile on his lips. Isa sleeps soundly in the baby sling he carries on his chest, her little face peeking out. Holding her close, he leans in to kiss my cheek tentatively. I notice an older woman in a doctor's coat as he steps back.

She beams at me, "Welcome back, love. I'm Dr. Radjeski." It's the British accent from my dream. Confused, I look at Colin.

"What's happening?" My throat is rough from disuse. Colin hesitates, glancing at the doctor. She takes the lead.

"You've successfully completed PASCUA, an extension of our deep brain stimulation program. This branch of our program treats those with what we call PASC, or post-acute sequelae SARS-CoV-2. Or, as it's commonly called, Long COVID. We enroll patients if medication and physical therapy are insufficient, when patients have given up."

I looked at Colin. He ran his hand over his beard. "Cam ... It's been over a year since you got COVID. You weren't getting better. The medicines just treated the symptoms. One day you were fine, and the next you'd crash, sometimes for days. You lost your job. You couldn't sleep. You were anxious and depressed. You tried to ..." His voice broke as he struggled to speak, "We got you to the hospital in time." He patted the sleeping baby as if she needed comfort.

I inhaled sharply, "I don't remember that part."

Colin clenched his fists and shook his head. "I should have seen it."

"No! You took care of me, took care of everyone." The corners of his mouth turned down, but he nodded.

The doctor stepped into the silence. "The hospital referred you to our program. Previously, we've used deep brain stimulation for conditions that show brain dysregulation: movement disorders, Parkinson's, obsessive-compulsive disorder, et cetera. We observed other positive side effects that allowed us to expand this treatment to Long COVID patients. It's an outpatient program, but it requires frequent return visits to customize the stimulation. Your care is, well, groundbreaking." She paused, allowing me to digest the information. My eyes cast around the room. Posy had moved to the floor to color in her storybook, her busy bag at her side. "By implanting electrodes in specific locations of your brain," she continued, "we stimulate the autonomic nervous system. The neurostimulator went under your collarbone. You may feel a slight bump there." I touched my collarbone but felt nothing. I closed my eyes, suddenly overwhelmed. My dream world beckoned.

No. I needed reality. My family. My life. I held tight to the present.

"By using your brain map, we can customize the stimulation. In layperson's terms, we're regulating your brain signals to improve your cardiovascular and respiratory function; normalizing blood pressure, orthostatic intolerance, breathing. Your experience varied because you've been here the whole time, asleep. The data flow is continuous."

"I slept the whole time?"

"Yes, you've been linked with this computer for four weeks," she patted the top of the monitor, "Its imagery program has directed your thoughts, allowing faster customization. We added an exciting enhancement to the imagery, partly owed to Colin. He mentioned you took up yoga. Consider this an intense guided meditation session to lower heart rate and blood pressure and increase oxygen. We accomplished in one month what normally takes well over four."

"Imagery program?"

"Highly personalized audio and video."

"Our trip to Japan," my brow wrinkled. "I couldn't move."

"Just imagery, to focus you inward. Planting the seed."

"My tree?"

“Yes, that’s the daily grounding meditation. A day isn’t enough time, so we chose a tree’s growth. Meditation helps, but we gloss over self-care, don’t we, love?”

I nodded.

“So, neurostimulation regulates the brainwave pattern. Neurofeedback trains your brain to generate and reinforce these patterns.” She smiled, “It’s time to go home. Enjoy your family, now. We’ll see you soon.”

West snored softly. Posy drew. Isa slept. “Ready?” Colin asks.

I looked at Posy. “Baby, what story was Daddy reading?”

Posy lifted the book. It showed a maiden sleeping in a castle. She’d drawn cherry blossoms around the margins. “Sleeping Beauty. It’s my favorite. Daddy says it’s your story.”

The Sinkhole

Kristy Malone

ESSAY

It's hard to express what Long COVID is like. Like all analogies, this is not a perfect one. It's based on an image that came to me in the midst of a debilitating flare. A flare that felt, to me, like an enormous pit of despair. The entire Long COVID experience feels a bit like that.

It's as if there's a giant, gaping sinkhole in the middle of a bustling city. To have Long COVID is to have fallen into the hole, unable to climb out of it. Reality shifts drastically, and our minds spin trying to make sense of it. We used to have access to the whole world and all its possibilities. Now the possibilities are limited to this small, shapeless space. We look up and see the sun make its way across the sky every day, but some corners of this sinkhole are so deep and cavernous that the sunlight never reaches them.

There is no clearly marked exit out of here. Some of us have been in the sinkhole for over three years; we know its terrain better than anyone. We've mapped every crevice and corner, and are now experts on something we never imagined we'd know this much about. Others have been here only a few weeks or months, still getting their bearings as the sinkhole veterans show them around.

Not everyone survives falling into the sinkhole of COVID-19. It has the power to claim lives. Millions, in fact, have been lost. We thought its lethality would cause people to regard the hole with respect, if not fear, but of course the official government narrative is that the hole only claims the lives of those who are old and going to die soon anyway or those who are unsteady on their feet and already prone to falling. A deadly sinkhole to an unlucky few, a mere pothole for the majority.

This is comforting to those who are neither old nor unsteady. It's been years now since the hole first appeared, and many now think of it as something in the past. Or they pretend it never existed at all. Any caution tape, fences, or warning signs have long been removed by officials, leaving no indications of threat. People don't want to be asked to live their lives differently just to protect others, especially if taking precautions would hurt the economy, limit freedoms, or cause stress.

Most people believe that they would never fall into a sinkhole. They think we must have done something wrong to be stuck down here. Or that we are just deeply unlucky. Or weak, or predisposed to falling. Or that it was our fear of the sinkhole itself that caused it to swallow us up. Or that it was our lack of faith in a higher power that left us vulnerable to falling. Such people have a higher power who would never let them fall, and what they don't fear and don't look at can't hurt them.

Others deny that we are in the hole at all. Peering down at us in disgust, they claim that the idea of being trapped is in our heads. We could climb out if we chose to. They speculate that we don't want to work, or that we seek attention. They don't stay long enough to hear our scream in response, "*No one* would choose to stay here if we had the ability to climb out!" The worst part about this particular group of people is that some were sent to help us

— trained experts in solving problems like this. They have years of education and impressive titles. The reality is that some experts would rather say that we're in a sinkhole of our own devising than admit that they don't know how to get us out.

Some of us in the sinkhole are lucky enough to have family and friends who reach down with supplies, a hand to hold, words of support. They remind us that we aren't forgotten, are still loved, still have value. They remind us that we still matter.

But we also have family and friends who turn their backs on us, who pretend the hole doesn't exist. Bewildered and feeling betrayed, we wonder how anyone could see what has become of us down here and ignore us? Simply continue with life as usual? As if there isn't this giant, gaping sinkhole indiscriminately swallowing people up every single day? Few are willing to accept the unpleasant reality that they too could fall in anytime.

Here in the sinkhole, our greatest resource is each other. People who never would have met before the sinkhole appeared now form a community here. Many of us were very different before falling in, but now we have so much in common. We find comfort here among the only people who can truly understand what we've all lost — here in this village of 65 million and growing. We tell each other, "You're not crazy. You're not lazy. You're stuck here, just like me." As in every village, there's some infighting. Being in the hole doesn't bring out the best of everyone. But it does bring out the best in some.

Who we were before we fell into the sinkhole is always on our minds. "I was a marathon runner," "A veterinarian," "I taught yoga three times a week," "A third grade teacher." Before, when we lived above ground, we had choices about who to be, how to use our time. Here, in the sinkhole, the choices we have are different. So we tell the story of who we used to be, what we used to do. So much of our identity was in doing, but down here it's in being. Being a person who can find humor in suffering, a person who makes another feel less alone, a person who can sit with difficult emotions, a person who keeps going when giving up is easier. We don't know whether to cling to the hope that we will return to our former selves, or accept our new identity as permanent. Few can understand what it's like to walk that painful knife's edge between hope and grief.

The sinkhole keeps expanding. It claims more victims every day. New arrivals say with bewilderment, "But I didn't know the sinkhole was still there!" Or "I didn't think it could happen to me!" They realize with shock that they are now a sinkhole dweller, largely invisible to the rest of the world. They demand answers. Why weren't they properly warned? Why wasn't a wall constructed around the sinkhole, or caution signs put up? Why isn't every news outlet reporting about the people in the sinkhole? Why aren't officials working around the clock to get us out? Why does the sinkhole continue to widen everyday, unchecked and largely ignored?

So many questions. So few answers.

Some people find their way out of the sinkhole after months or years. Some of them never look back, while others take the time to explain how they escaped, so that others might get out too. We haven't found a way out that works for everyone, but we've learned more from each other than we have from anyone on the ground level about how to escape.

Those of us who have been in the sinkhole long enough have gained a new perspective on life. Down here in the dark, we find parts of ourselves that we couldn't see as well in the sunlight. There's so much to discover in the absence of all that "doing." From here, we can now see the other sinkholes people had fallen into before, that we never saw before. Or maybe we saw them but assumed someone else would help the people stuck at the bottom. We certainly never thought a sinkhole could swallow *us* up, or that help wouldn't come if it did.

We realize that even if we get out of this hole eventually, we'll never be the same. We'll never see the world or the people in it the same way. In some ways that is a good thing, and we're grateful. There's so much we won't take for granted again. In other ways, we grieve the people we were before we understood the reality of the sinkholes all around us, and the people who pass right by them without a thought.

There are some above ground who see the sinkhole for the crisis it is. They understand that anyone could fall into the hole, and that many more are destined to do just that. They warn others but are often dismissed, even mocked. It takes courage to focus on the problem that no one wants to look at. It's a curious thing that in one context saving lives is applauded as heroic, but in another it's ridiculed. The rescue is so complex, and there are so many people down here it will require a large-scale, coordinated effort among experts from many disciplines. Their efforts give us hope, but the problem seems to grow faster than the rescuers can mobilize.

Many questions remain. Will the sinkhole eventually swallow the entire planet and everyone who lives on it? Will we all become sinkhole people, and maybe one day forget that there was a time we lived above ground? Will the rest of our lives be spent in the hole finding whatever comfort or peace we can, or is there another chapter of our stories that will take place above ground? Will enough people take action and work together to warn the public, stabilize the sinkhole, and pull the survivors out? For now, we make a home here in this village of uncertainty. We focus on being instead of doing. We light candles where the sunlight doesn't reach. And we wait.

My Life on the Long Haul

Nikki Stewart

ESSAY

I am always tired. Never not tired. My life changed suddenly, drastically, and irrevocably in December 2020. I'm a survivor, and I thank God every day that I'm still here — that I got off the oxygen — and that I could return to my 9-to-5. While I'm a survivor, I'm not yet a thriver. And I'm tired.

My deficits, my wounds, if you will, are not visible. They are not obvious or tangible; worse, they are not quantifiable: *You look OK? You must be OK. I mean, you look so much better than you did before. Maybe you just need more exercise? You should go to bed earlier. You don't need that handicapped placard. I mean, you're just tired.*

My brain is foggy on a good day, with many words dancing out of reach. I loved words once. They were my friends. Now they hide from me, waiting, hoping I'll find them. They know there is a good chance I never will. Not while they matter. Maybe later. Maybe. Words and thoughts slip out of my head like sand through my fingers. From one sentence to the next — from one second to the next — I don't know what I was saying or thinking. Where was I going with this? Focus! Don't forget about focus. It's hard to focus. Maybe I'll find that later, too. But not while I'm tired.

My life is a series of managed moments, matching tasks to time and energy. My stamina is limited. Things waiting to be done feel infinite. I personify a sixth grade math problem as I do the calculations: if I do X activity for Y amount of time, how long will I need to rest to recover? Will I have the time to recover? I have to factor in the constant, that is, the 9-to-5. I need time to recover from the job. Perhaps I'll put off activity X until next week, but I have to do the cooking, cleaning, or laundry one of these weeks. Thank goodness for Instacart. It's a blessing for people who are tired.

Let's not forget the job, with all its demands that start before 9 and never end at 5. I train my community — teach them how to stay healthy, tell them how early detection of cancer saves lives. I educate while losing words. I make health presentations without the energy to be present. I meet them where they are, church, school, social clubs — any day, anytime, all the while trying not to look like I am tired.

Sometimes I miss the little things. Things I never knew helped me find connection. Something I never knew helped to ground me, like communing with nature on a walk through the park preserve, enveloped by the blanket of greenery, or spending a day at a music festival, my heart matching the beat of the jazz and funk. Things like dancing in my beloved's arms, knowing this is the place I was born to be. Now, I sit on benches as others walk by. Now I go to concerts in the park for an hour. Now I watch my beloved dance, wishing I could join in. I do these things when I can, when the calculations work out, and when I'm not too tired.

But there is grace in the long haul. Not so long ago, but in the before — the before when I walked, the before when I danced — I lived and died by a calendar packed to bursting. I raced from pillar to post, activity to event, ensuring I was everywhere. Making sure I disappointed no one. I could do it all if I tried hard and raced fast enough. Maybe doing all of that would make me good enough. So I ran, trying to keep up with a life full of demands and obligations, barely taking time for walks, seldom giving up whole days for festivals, and rarely dancing with my beloved. Now that I manage and calculate, I choose the moments that matter. Now I know there is power in saying "No." I also know now that before, I was already tired.

And so I learn. I learned the lessons I knew before. I realize the things children know instinctively: take care of myself first. I also listen to my body and mind. Making time for self-care doesn't mean I'll lose the race. Saying I have had enough doesn't mean *I'm* not enough.

Most of all, I have learned the importance of my village, and the people who raise me up, and keep me going. These people showed me the power of strength in numbers and didn't wait for me to ask for help. They taught me that I am enough. That I don't have to be OK, and I am enough. That my thoughts can drift away, and I am enough.

I may be tired, but I am enough.

today today today

Christopher Soden

it was better today i thought to cook
macaroni and cheese with butter
and condensed milk and drove chloe
to the park where i sat on a shiny
painted blue wooden bench and let her

wander the length of the leash while i
took refuge in shades and black
surgical mask why havent i got any
stamina lately my knees and ankles ache
my neck is heavy i was raised by television

and watch for hours and make inane gags
and talk to mother knowing she is content
and vigilant and soaring on the far side
of the veil i welcome the spectacle
of lightning drumming and rolling and smile

to comfort my familiars (though i wonder
if benevolent imperialism is humane)
and the rain is lovely when im settled in
my grandad used to say it was crucial to leave
the house at least once every day

for any reason you could find mailing
a letter or getting ice cream or circling
the lake it still helps to find something
truly defiant on the car radio i write now
to a casual friend who shares accounts

of impulsive sexual episodes though
hes not as intrepid as he sounds
finding another guy in the woods
who spits to make penetration
less excruciating but i still write back

i believe a routine (long shower
fresh bright island shirts cologne
two hours refining my poems)
would help rid me of this persistent
queasiness this dull thumping headache
this dread of something inexplicable

will i ever salvage my furious
sister will i have soap for laundry
what will i smear on sardines
will i reconcile with my also dead
father the starving bully i need

the crush of someone without grace
someone who will soothe me
with moist banana and dark red
pintos someone that will kiss me
without terror someone that wont
stop sobbing

Naive Optimism

May Patiño

Nearly 25 years before my Long COVID journey began, I went on my first solo road trip. I was 18 years old. I ended up driving through a blizzard.

Over the years, I have found myself reflecting on this experience, realizing, in waves, how influential it has been in shaping who I am today. I have often wondered, if I had known that trip would have been such a disaster, would I still have gone? In that same vein, if we knew then what we know now about Long COVID, would we have handled the pandemic differently?

ESSAY

When I pulled onto the interstate, the slightest mist of snow was falling. No chain requirements were posted, so it didn't seem ominous. As I started up the mountainous incline, the snow slowly grew heavier and heavier. But there were still cars on the road, so I carried on, unconcerned.

The snow kept thickening. It turned out the pass had been closed 10 minutes after I had gotten on the interstate. Had I known, I'm sure I would have turned around. This could have been the end of the story if I had seen a warning sign.

Semitrucks began pulling off to the shoulder. Then, one after another, I watched as cars slid off the road, jamming their brakes. Terrified to tap on mine, I downshifted and followed the taillights before me. The snow was building up on my windshield, making it harder and harder to see. Eventually, my windshield wipers couldn't even move.

Snow continued to fall, and soon, everything went very quiet. I could no longer tell if there were other cars on the road. To see anything, I had to scrunch my head down to the steering wheel's height. Only a three-inch gap remained uncovered by the snow. I kept my head down, peering out my peephole, driving at five miles an hour and not daring to touch my brakes until I saw the exit on the other side of the pass. I was too frightened to stop until then.

When I pulled into town, the snowfall stopped. It was much later than I anticipated, but there was still a sliver of daylight, so I took deep breaths and found a gas station. I filled up my tank, to calm my nerves more than anything. When I turned back onto the street, in a momentary lapse of awareness, I tapped my brakes and found myself sliding until I hit the curb. Knowing what I know now, this is where the story could have ended.

The interstate was quiet and clear. I was steadily making my way south, feeling relieved that this next leg of my trip would be smoother. I figured I'd probably reach my destination in time for a late dinner. After an hour, though, traffic suddenly stopped. I was still 30 miles from the next city. The snowfall had returned, and soon, engines started to shut off. I followed suit and abruptly realized this meant no more heat. If I hadn't kept a comforter in the trunk of my car, this could have been the end of the story. But I did (who doesn't?), so it wasn't. I bundled up and hunkered down until past dark. I was still waiting, hoping for a sign of movement. I only saw a sea of cars on all sides.

Minutes turned to hours. Empty stomach rumbles turned to loud, angry growls. Finally, just over four hours later, we all rejoiced when traffic started moving. Then, suddenly, just as the city lights came into view, my car completely died right in the middle of the freeway.

I was alone and stranded in pitch dark and before the time of cellphones. Terrified that I would get run into by oncoming traffic at any moment, my mind bounced between panic and logic. My hazard lights blinked until a patrol car eventually pulled behind me with the promise of a midnight tow truck and a ride to the closest motel. I was told I would have to take my car to the shop in the morning.

Ten hours after leaving home, on what was supposed to be a five-hour journey, this was only just my halfway point. I remember having the foresight to get a debit card before I left home. I was excited and scared to use it for the first time when I paid for the motel room. I ordered a pizza and breathed a sigh of relief, an immense wave of exhaustion washing over me.

Suddenly, there was a knock at my door. Startled, I walked over to it, thinking the pizza guy must have forgotten something. But I didn't recognize this man I saw on the other side of the door. He wasn't the pizza guy, motel staff, or tow truck driver. He said nothing; he just kept knocking. I shook like a leaf and crumpled into a ball on the motel room floor, scrunched up against the foot of the bed. He knocked, knocked, knocked. Then silence. Then knock, knock, knock. Silence. Knock. Repeat. It went on for minutes that felt like eons. This could have been the end of the story, too. Finally, I heard footsteps walking away. I'll never know who it was or what they wanted, but I know they didn't stop at anyone else's door. In the morning, I took my car to an auto shop. It turned out my starter was broken.

I think back to this trip often since COVID and, subsequently, Long COVID came along to turn my life upside down. I can now see how I approached COVID with the same naive optimism I did that storm. I had been sick before, so surely I would be fine after this. COVID just felt like a light snow flurry. In the beginning, Long COVID felt like peering through a peephole in my windshield: I could still see daylight. My destination was ever onward, more important than any momentary fear. So, I continued onward through my new snowy conditions, not knowing how to survive any other way. It felt too dangerous to tap on the breaks of my life, to stop working. Back then, I was still driving at close to normal speeds, feeling at times almost fully recovered despite signs of a brewing storm. Powering through, after all, is what we are always told to do.

Then, one day, four months after my Long COVID journey began, my starter suddenly went kaput. I was bedridden for three months and still housebound more than a year later. In the beginning, during those bedridden nights, I would often wake with a jolt: The anxiety I experienced with Long COVID wasn't like any I had ever felt before, and it terrified me just as much as a stranger knocking on my motel room door.

If I had known then what I know now, I wouldn't have returned to work until I fully recovered. I would have known that stroke-like symptoms, bouts of debilitating fatigue, crippling nerve pain, and worsening brain fog meant *stop*. Work should never have to take priority over health. I can't help but imagine what life might be like for me and the millions of others with Long COVID if we had broad public health campaigns, clearly and loudly letting people know about the hazards. Will we ever be capable of collectively deciding to avoid driving headlong into a storm?

When I think of this trip, I think of it as my reminder to remain calm in times of crisis and to watch and listen for the small and nuanced warning signs. It's a reminder that sometimes you must embrace the tough-as-nails fearlessness of a naive teenager when life hurls unprecedented times at you. If I could navigate that treacherous storm, then I've got this challenge. Long COVID could be the end of my story, but it's not. It's a reminder that I've always been a survivor. We are all survivors.

Rusted Out

Adrienne Asher

Like a chainsaw that won't pull,
my lungs grind out attempts
at starting up, and fail.
I put my shoulder into it
and cough, grab a few breaths,
choke, then start up breathing.
Walking on legs shaky
as a newborn colt, I totter
to the kitchen, hellbent on arrival.
Head dizzied, joints aching,
I make black tea strong
as last night's fever.

Before Coffee, Before Food

Adrienne Asher

The woman with cobweb hair skips
bathing when the fever screams,
sits down fast, writes faster. Thinks
out loud, always reads poetry barefoot,
except in winter, when it's hiking boots.
Keeps a weather eye on the spaces
between fenceposts, crafts hashtags
like tech haiku, parenthetical rap
on global buzz. She is made from
the pieces of her life she remembers,
the rest is marginalia, red-lined by a virus
too deadly to remember, too hot to name.
Writing in a flurry, in a fury, she meets silence.
One mile from hope, the lights fade out.

Once, He Went Out Dancing

Adrienne Asher

My lungs ache like I've been kicked
breathless by some Puget Sound logger's
leather boots. I feel the imprint of lug soles,
know he's put some muscle into it
after a long night, drunk and chain-smoking,
trying to outrun one bad marriage
and three young kids. He won't recover
anytime soon. I will, but still, this damned
cough won't stop, won't let me rest,
and I'm not made for barroom brawls.

Flee as a Bird to Your Mountain

Adrienne Asher

As all the birds, singing, stop
when danger creeps along the ground,
just so, my lungs, filled with a viral damage,
try pumping but then hesitate.

The scents of cigarette and wood smoke
drift through my midnight rooms, phantoms
no one else can sense. I have become
a word spoken by solitude and silence,

punctuated by explosive coughs,
held within the journal of a devouring
thing that moves and morphs
more quickly than my hand can write.

So my March eyes (not water, not snow),
gray winter eyes, street-slushed,
blink dryly, watching tilting stars
count out this long night's hours.

Certain People

Sonya Huber

ESSAY

We wave to Mizzy every day we see him inside the barbershop, cutting mostly Black men's hair at the seat closest to the door. We walk down Main Street with our goofy dog, who summons chicken bones and hunks of God knows what from the sidewalk. Mizzy gives not a New England nod nor a fainthearted flip of the fingers but a dazzling smile you can see even around his mask, eyes alight through his glasses, and a full-body wave that animates his lanky frame.

We walk past the Dunkin' Donuts, then wave to the woman who sells us Chinese food. She nods shyly. A few shops down is the stylist where my husband, Cliff, goes to get his hair cut, and when we pass, we wave to the two women inside. After a haircut one day, Cliff came home to tell me that his haircut lady told him Mizzy was in the hospital with COVID-19 and that it got complicated because he also had MS.

I'd seen his cane in the way that a cane is a language, a bond. Its metal curve mirrored the one I used on days when my rheumatoid arthritis stabbed and nipped. Knowing that Mizzy was in a hospital bed slipped into my flesh briefly, hit me in the chest. I felt it forward and backward in time, readjusting what I knew of Mizzy, reimagining the devastation I knew of COVID-19 when it powered into you: the fever, the dry cough, and then the needling into the brain, the heart, the vessels; the way it colonized and hungered for your entire landscape. We glanced into the barbershop every day as we passed, waiting for Mizzy to reappear behind the plate glass at the first chair.

Our daily walks with the dog were a kind of parade route for me, a more precious and urgent pacing these days. I got COVID-19 in March 2020 during the lockdown — always an early adopter of the latest technology. Then came six months of being unable to even walk around the block without being destroyed the next day, gasping for breath with heart damage, lung spots, a brain frazzled, and sleep destroyed. Thank God for my fellow long haulers who made Slack groups and text chains, who documented and shared stories, theories, and ideas for treatments in a furious explosion — all while severely ill — that laid the foundation for everything we know about the syndrome. We saved each other and did first-person research remotely while seriously ill. We saved some of us. We made knowledge from our beds and are making it still.

After six terrifying months, I got better, as in more able to walk, but I'll never be the same. I have post-exertional malaise and an "energy envelope" to stay inside. It is an envelope with a window I can see through, like Mizzy in his window.

I feel the stares and awkwardness of friends who read fear onto me because I'm still masking, though they should be reading the savvy cool of someone who's stared at the skull of death and continued to function. I feel a coldness surrounding me. People who say they care about me judge my mask and write that I am a mouthless cipher. I am no longer invited to events and hangouts. The full warmth and urgency only return when they need me, when well people — privately shocked to have a chronic condition — message me and others with Long COVID: *Tell me what to do; how do I exist now*? I am an object for them, a compass or a map. They don't admit their syndromes in the windows of social media.

Then, one day, Mizzy reappears in the window. We see him and wave with our whole bodies, two-handed emphatic joyful waves, and he comes outside (my place now, my ventilated heaven of safety) to see us. It turns out he is the sweetest possible person, and we say we are so glad to see him and that the hair ladies down the street told us what had happened.

Mizzy tells us he thinks it might be a government conspiracy, this virus, and in a way, he's entirely correct: it is the state, the entire power structure of inequality mapped here, that visits risk on those who are not white, who do not have money, who do not have privilege. One recent medical study says that "certain people" are more likely to get Long COVID. Which group? Women are twice as likely. Double. Other "certain people" include people of color, those who weigh more, those with autoimmune conditions, and those with depression. Who is left out of these circles? The study presents this as "good news and bad news." What the hell, pardon my French, is the upside? The virus enters the body, encountering its immune system vaults of multigenerational memory, and the body grapples with a space alien, an utterly foreign object.

I don't think the virus is a conspiracy, but I understand the deep vein beneath what Mizzy says and connect to it in the gut of my being. "It's something different, right?" I ask. "It feels like nothing you've ever felt before." Mizzy turns toward me, not only with his head but his torso and hips, the way our knowledge of our entire bodies has shifted.

"Right?" he says. "You have to respect it."

Then Mizzy says, "I like you guys. It makes me happy to see you every day." He tells my husband and me that he could tell by looking at us that we weren't from around here, that he likes that. My husband and I, prone to full-body laughter, look at each other and laugh.

We walk down the street past the old gas station that is being turned into something new, and I say, "Conspiracy...," not in amusement but trying to feel my way into that reality. When my husband says, "I'd much rather hear that than 'It's just a cold,'" I agree.

"Just a cold" is the complete denial, the seamless fantasy, the true conspiracy of silence.

And Mizzy, in his window most days, still wears a mask to cut hair, and he waves as if this day is given but not guaranteed, and I wave back.

A Possible Last Testament from a Long COVID Survivor

Brian Burke

ESSAY

When I first heard about an anthology of stories by people with Long COVID, I was excited but unsure what to write. Stories about COVID-19 from a few artists and writers inspire me, and after much thinking, I decided to share my story and my mother's.

I have been close to death many times. Becoming sick with COVID-19 in 2021 was another dire close call. But while I survived, my mother, Teresa Burke, did not. The loss of my mother has brought continuing physical and mental pain. Everything is much worse now than before COVID-19. I thought I would be doing better by now, but I may not live much longer.

I should tell you about life before COVID. I was born autistic in 1978, but in early childhood, doctors did not know what I had and gave me the wrong medication and treatment, sometimes making me very sick. I did not receive a correct diagnosis until the 1990s.

In that same era, I was violently attacked and threatened and had to leave the school and town I grew up in. The trauma from it was so severe that I attempted suicide twice, first in 1997 and then again later. I still have PTSD from the violence. Some days are better than others, though, and recently, I have begun to feel I have a new purpose.

By the 2000s, I developed a heat sensitivity, making me susceptible to heat illness and severe heat strokes. My body is 20 degrees hotter than the temperature. The hotter the weather, the worse it gets, and a 90-degree day feels like 110 degrees. In 2006, my mom nursed me back to health by consulting with doctors and ensuring I drank lots of electrolyte drinks.

People need to know that long haulers want to work. Over the years, it has been hard to get a job, and the few I did get were usually through disability agencies. At most jobs, they don't want me around much due to my disabilities, yet these agencies offer protection from that. So many agencies are closed down now, post-COVID, or have severely limited staff.

In 2007, a nearly four-year stretch began where our housing was unstable. First, my mother and I were evicted and became homeless when we lacked enough rent money. She moved around a bit, and I stayed with my father. After that, through 2010, Mom and I stayed in motels, with family, and in our car. At one point, the heat inside the car was so bad that I once again almost died from heatstroke. Our family and friends helped when they could, and in 2011, we moved into a new apartment where I still live.

In the 1990s, I started making, selling, and exhibiting T-shirts, magazines, and films but only brought in a little money. My mother took art classes before I was born. Then, in 2011, she developed a new love of painting. Over the next decade, she created over 100 pieces and exhibited some. We both got a lot out of the People's Resource Center classes, where a teacher named Lesley Gena changed my mother's life. Today, I continue to make art in Mom's memory and am trying to sell her works.

We carefully avoided getting COVID-19. Things changed in February

2021 when I had COVID-19 pneumonia symptoms soon after visiting a store. A few days later, things became a blur as we spent most of our time on the bathroom or kitchen floor, lying in our waste, sometimes trying to stand up only to fall, badly and repeatedly. I apologize for being gross, but it is the truth. I later learned from medical people that we had damaged both the floor and our bodies, which worsened our conditions.

At some point, I called 911. The paramedics helped us get into the ambulance. I was given many medications in the hospital, including steroids, and then sent home after a few days because it was overcrowded. Once home, I turned off all the lights we left on. I was still so sick that cleaning things up took over a week. Little by little, I started to get better.

My mother transferred to different facilities where some people abused and robbed her. In April 2021, she came home and seemed to be getting better as I helped care for her. Yet, within a week, she had a seizure due to COVID-19 damage and a foot infection. She returned to the hospital and then went into hospice. She could communicate only on and off.

She passed away on June 13, 2021, just before her birthday.

Mom wanted to be cremated and made me promise to wait before holding her memorial to give people a break. Some relatives continue to help, and I am fundraising on GoFundMe and planning a memorial that will include videos and a display of her art. Since her death, my health has worsened, and I can barely survive with a cut or reduction in disability benefits. I used to want to die, but now I want to live, mainly to keep that one promise.

My daily reality is a nightmare. I might fall asleep quickly each night but then wake up two hours later. I struggle to fall back asleep, even with the help of medication, and often lie down, barely able to move, wanting to sleep. Usually, I cannot. So I just lay there, feeling like I am barely alive.

Basic things like going to the store or library are now so exhausting I have to lie down when I get home, if I even get home before collapsing somewhere. Most jobs want people for fast food or heavy lifting, which I can't do. My community and family still contact me but have their struggles. I have lost many jobs and continually experience a lot of chest and stomach pain. My breathing is still terrible, and I may have a stress ulcer. I'm taking medications, but getting to medical testing and treatments is challenging because my transportation program has been cut and is no longer free.

I was in an online therapy program to help with PTSD and the loss of my mother, but the therapist dropped me without warning or reason. There seemed to be no other therapists available for weeks. Online COVID-19 and NAMI (National Alliance on Mental Illness) groups offer some support, but it's tough to function. I am not emotionally well and have PTSD flares. I recently started with a new therapist, so that's good news. A computer is vital for many activities and work-at-home jobs. My laptop computer recently stopped operating. Traveling to a charity that fixes computers for free may be challenging.

If I don't have much time left, I hope people will remember me as someone who tried to do what my mother asked. I may have failed her just like I failed at so much else. I try to fix things and would apologize if I knew what I did wrong, but most of the time, people don't tell me what I did wrong. How can I improve if no one tells me what I did wrong? A person can only take so much, but I continue to make art, videos, and books.

Some horrible events happened to my mother, and she almost killed herself. One day in 1982, she broke down crying because her mother's cancer worsened. Even though I was only 3, I walked over and patted her with my hand as if to say, "It's OK. There, there," like I had seen others do. It also comforted her just to watch me sleeping. Toward the end of her life, we talked about how much I meant to her and how I'd saved her life. She said, "I love you," and asked that I please promote her artwork, which I keep doing. Yet I wonder as I get sicker and am in more pain: if I did save her all those years ago, then what is my purpose now?

Thank you for listening to my story.

Outside the civil war

Morgan Stephens

The body against the body,
me fighting me,
for me,
infantry lining up,
steady, steady,
no need to be briefed,
like the fineness of my father's hair
turned my hair,
we charge forward in a losing war.

Outside, where land meets sea,
I have grown gentle,
the kind that comes with loss, of knowing,
broken in by what decay can do.

I look out at stained spaces,
pillowgazed, I glimpse
suburban creatures, scurrying
through their large little lives.

I look out
at all the lobbies,
in all the cities,

we tick in the waiting rooms
and bury our hands in bags
to find our bottle for this one.
They have gentleness, too, taken,
tucked behind skin.

To know that among the daggers,
underneath the casting off
death, inevitable, not today but
one day,
one day,
we wrestle with a fragile sword.

But outside the civil war,
I am softened,
the ruin of illness has
mellowed me, reddish brown
as the cinnamon in my tea,
the birds and the squirrels
live on,
blessed not knowing their fate.

The only pandemic daughter

Morgan Stephens

The first-born daughter
That makes me the eldest daughter
Yet you have got two brothers to protect you daughter
The never saw them again daughter
The left holding the bag daughter
The only one who showed up daughter
The one to get a degree daughter
The no trophy photos daughter
The quarantine in a hotel to cover president's daughter
The heard my name yelled daughter
The saw my father convulsing daughter
The time to do what you do best daughter
The make the call, talk to the paramedics daughter
Stay back, we all have COVID, daughter
The thumping, pulse-racing, chasing down daughter
The calm, steady, steady, steady now, daughter
The I got it, I'll take care of it daughter
The my coffee tastes funny, metallic daughter
The I'm just stressed, work to the bone daughter
The tough-as-nails trope daughter
It found its way into you anyway daughter

The trembling, 3 a.m., am I having a stroke daughter
Hallway tilted, YouTube ASMR, pass the time daughter
I don't know if I'm going to survive this daughter
In the gray mist morning, father says
"Remember where you came from," widowed
grandmother's granddaughter
But I never knew her much I think daughter
Wailing, naked, body does not belong to me anymore
daughter
Mother-washed hair by a plastic stadium cup daughter
The screamed in that house for sixty days daughter
Can we put her in a coma, he asked, daughter
The leaving, forced smile, I'll be OK, daughter
She tried to end her life phone call daughter
The cold, silver dishwasher "No," moaning daughter.
The get on a plane no matter what daughter
The everything will be OK daughter
The hide the sharp objects in a cooler next-door daughter
In the psych ward she looked tiny and frail daughter
My lion of a mother turned mouse daughter
If I get healthy again, we'll try for a baby daughter
She could have the same eyes as you daughter
The heir to who looks over with sympathy, to
The sullen boy in visiting hours daughter
Her eyes crinkle and whisper

"He's schizophrenic" daughter
The one who barely knows her family daughter
The one who knows them best daughter
The one who does not know where she came from daughter
It lives inside her neurotransmitters instead daughter
Burning dignity, yearning to live or die daughter
My mother's, mother's, mother's daughter

A bath on Christmas Day

Morgan Stephens

Sundry swirl sherbet
of sunset, creamsicle,

sting my bones, numb and sigh
out loud, to the pine

soft yuletide, mute the streets
soapy slosh of steam

where hold-on season found me,
I get up shimmering,

the chrysalis deserted,
clean.

The body and the palm

Morgan Stephens

California gave me her grace
again, to return
in sunlight and heat
slanted against my broken body,
in lavender and sea salt
sticking sweetly to thinning hair,
daffodils in spring,
sprouting against the sterile
year of winter hospitals
in windowless blue gowns
where I gave over my abandoned body
and possessions
to the masks
as they handed out sandpaper-yellow socks.

Back to inroads
that wind and stop and go
without permission,
veins that dilate, bulging blue
deep in the sun-drenched valleys
of tendon and bone,
marking
that this is not over,

a vessel by me to me
into the upright palm
that sways and shades
the catastrophe,
abundant in her season,
I look up to find her once again.

Endurance

Morgan Stephens

nobody can tell me
when the haunt retreats
not the doctors—
the first one
or the fifty-fourth
my pain specialist
or my neurologist
my immunologist
or my hypnotist
not mother
or father
Jerry
or Anne

none can tell me
how long I will
wake up
sideways
blurred out
leadlimbed
stuck in the dusk wheel

She had so much promise.
It's sad, really.

nobody can tell me when this ends
when the light starts peeling
the cold wind off my face
nobody can tell me
how much of me is gone
buried and rotting under flesh
as I slowly retreat
and fungus crawls

A new, unknown illness.
A casualty.
A shame.

nobody can tell me when this ends
it's up to me to feel it
my gut to know it
my body to sense it

nobody can tell me when this ends
I step on the sidewalk
do what it tells me, and tilt.

The Smell of Farts and Desperation

Nina Storey

ESSAY

This is not a story about COVID. This story is about when I adopted a dog while recovering from Long COVID. You get to decide which has been more stressful.

Four months after getting sick, I adopted a dog with as many medical issues as I have. This was not on purpose. Good Lord, the last thing I would have wanted while recovering from COVID is a dog needing more medical attention than me.

I thought a dog would mean unconditional love and cuddling and, yes, an occasional poop in the living room. And also sometimes, he would go to the bathroom in the house. But I think I got catfished by the dog formerly known as "Inmate Number 799."

Inmate, or "Bubsie," as I now call him, had an online profile describing him as "perfect," "petite," and an "absolute angel." But when I walked through the doors of the animal rescue to see this 70-pound, four-legged terrorist destroying a full-sized rubber tire, I realized his Instagram presence was as airbrushed as an advertisement for butt-lifting leggings.

When I got him home, I realized I'd adopted either a raging hypochondriac or a dog competing to see which of us could score more visits to the emergency room. For those of you counting, we're each logged in at five apiece.

On the other hand, maybe all of his medical conditions were him attempting to get closer to me. Perhaps I should have, instead, called them sympathy ailments:

Skin rash and losing hair. I got that too.

Eye infection. Ditto.

Sinus problems. You betcha.

Autoimmune issue. Me too! Here, take my prescription for doxycycline. I'm done with it.

Prone to yeast infections. I hear that, sister!

Can't eat carbs because it causes inflammation. Both of us are lamenting life without cookies.

After spending an embarrassing amount of my money on what would have been my dream vacation to Tahiti, Bubsie then had to take ungodly expensive nutritional supplements and could eat only dehydrated meat and freshly steamed vegetables. No offense, and please don't hate me, but fuck thisgoddamneddog.

Every morning for months, I dragged my lethargic COVID-19 ass out of bed to make him a fried egg, fresh steamed broccoli, and rehydrate a bowl of gruel that looked like canned World War II rations. As a result, my apartment perpetually smelled like farts and desperation.

In the darkest part of my illness, my body did not have the strength to even lift my head off the pillow, and things like showering felt like an Olympic sport reserved for those with the bicep endurance of Serena Williams. To keep my blood pressure from perpetually tanking, I often had to salt my water, my potato chips, and on occasion, my armpits. And I'd be lying to say I didn't drink regularly from the pickle jar. Often I wouldn't have the energy to brush my teeth, yet I would simultaneously feel like my heart had been tethered to the saddle of an angry rodeo bull. It felt like my body was shouting, "Hurry up and drop dead already!"

There were a lot of days my dog didn't get the exercise he needed. But he loyally served as my knee pillow and fart dampener, rarely complaining. And as long as I kept feeding him his gruel, he stayed close by my side. I'm guessing it had to have been a bummer for him too. He finally gets adopted after surviving months on the mean streets of Bakersfield, only to now be living life as a couch cushion. I don't exactly think this was his idea of leveling up.

So it makes perfect sense that his spirits had been diminished throughout this experience. I even noticed he resorted to day drinking. This would also explain what happened to all my emergency water.

At times when my ability to take care of myself was hanging by a thread, speaking words became painfully difficult. I spent days in silence, mind racing to understand this waking prison I barely existed in. My feet felt like loaded sandbags, and merely stepping outside to let Bubsie pee took all the strength I could muster.

I'm guessing if you're a giant cattle dog, that has to be a bit of a buzz kill. Five measly minutes outside has got to be its own sort of personal hell too. So one night, when I walked into the living room to find him lying on the couch next to an open bottle of pills, I couldn't help but think, *Well, one of us was bound to do it.*

At the stroke of midnight, there he was trying to Marilyn Monroe himself. What was I supposed to do? I had no idea what he'd taken, how much of it, and, more importantly, why? I know he didn't mean to swallow that bottle of pills but it's hard not to take it personally, especially considering I found a note reading, "Woof. Also, it's all your fault."

He obviously didn't leave a handwritten note. He's illiterate. But he was telling me something. Perhaps he was just trying to get me to watch something other than hours upon hours of *Star Trek*. Maybe he was simply trying to get to the unwrapped Jolly Rancher stuck to the bottom of my purse. Whatever the reason, two things were certain: 1. I now had to rush him to the hospital to have his stomach pumped. 2. He knew how to use a zipper.

So even though my body felt like lead dropped to the bottom of a swimming pool and I was rocking a mild case of vertigo, I drove him to the vet where they quickly induced vomiting. Resting my body against the nearest wall to keep the ground from becoming the ceiling, I thought "Am I a bad pet owner? How was I to know he could unzip a bag without thumbs?"

Fifteen minutes later, the doctor stepped out onto the sidewalk holding a giant rubber container filled with the contents of my dog's stomach.

"What do you think?" he asked me.

"I can't say for sure, because I'm not a doctor, but I'm guessing this is a tub full of throw-up."

"Yeah, that's what we think too." *Really? This is why they charged me $600?* Here I was being forced to put my nose into his vomit. Shouldn't I have shit in someone's shoe to deserve this kind of treatment?

"We just want to be sure you recognize what's in his stomach. Also, we don't see any pills. But to be on the safe side, we should pump him full of more medication because he could die from . . ." and then his voice became like the adults in every Charlie Brown cartoon. All I could hear was squawking and muted vowel sounds. I then slowly handed over my bank card and politely asked him to remove the vomit trough from my face.

Four hours and two emergency room visits later, he was getting treated for a laundry list of concerns and was staying the night. I drove my weary body home and slept harder than I had in weeks.

The next morning I felt unusually refreshed. Maybe it was the barf-infused aromatherapy or just that the burden of having to take care of another sickly creature in addition to myself had been temporarily lifted, but it was the closest thing to a vacation I'd taken in over two years. So that morning I hunkered down and I cradled my pillow with the affection of a drunken college student embracing a warm pizza pie.

I slept through the day into the evening until the animal hospital called to say my dog probably didn't have any pills still in his system, but they were keeping him another day just to be safe. They assured me he was getting walked four times a day, eating fresh chicken, receiving daily massages, and was overall, in good spirits. That's when I had the thought: *thatgoddamnedgod did it on purpose.*

So while my dog remained at his five-star day spa, I retreated back to my medically induced staycation. The floor became lava and I had no reason to leave my tugboat, I mean bed, for the next 24 hours.

When I picked Bubsie up the next day, he had a spring in his step, a bow on his neck and he cried saying goodbye to the armed security guard holding the door.

Since his return home, this adorable nugget with excessive chin fat has continued to be a source of love and aggravation for me. While the hospital resuscitated his will to live, he now takes extraordinary joy in imitating the running of the bulls whenever the mood suits him. Without intention or malice, he's accidentally tripped me well over a dozen times using mostly illegal football tackles, given me one black eye, injured both my knees, forced me to eat a pavement sandwich twice, and consistently failed to protect me from spraying skunks, aggressive canines or humans, and meandering house spiders.

Thankfully, through all of this though, the one thing that has slowly improved, is me. After three-plus years of rehab and fistfuls upon fistfuls of both Western and Eastern medicine, I am starting to get better.

My endurance is stronger, I can walk farther, and I can do that thing where you shower, make breakfast, drive places, and brush your teeth before bed. I don't want to brag, but who has two thumbs, a driver's license, and a Safeway card? Yep, Thumbs McGee even recently went shopping in a grocery store for the first time in eight months! I'm taking the tiny wins as giant victories and lemme tell you, picking out my own tampons ranks high among them.

While I am still in treatment for Long COVID symptoms and some days I feel like I've been pushed into a barrel of tar that's been thrown into a bathtub along with a plugged-in toaster, I'm focused on taking it one day at a time. I'm working hard to appreciate the little things, like a long breath of fresh air without chest pain, or walking my giant, dopey dog down the block, while I follow closely behind picking up his dinosaur-sized poops with a shopping cart.

In the new times, it's hard to say what is normal, and I think I lost my membership to normalcy the day I decided to like pineapple and mayonnaise sandwiches. So instead, I've decided to relish both the days when I feel like a baggie full of jelly, and also the days I can twirl around my living room with my pre-COVID joie de vivre. Each now has precious value in my world.

The Struggle Is Real

Corie Mogenis

ESSAY

I never imagined that I would become terribly ill when the pandemic hit. In March 2020, I suddenly had every symptom on the news detailing this new virus. Doctors reassured me that I had bronchitis and should "calm down" and stop watching TV. My chest X-ray was clear, so even though I couldn't breathe, coughed nonstop, and had zero energy or voice, they said not to worry. It took me two months to start to feel normal again.

In July, I started feeling very strange one day. Within minutes, I was slurring my words, tingling, and shaking uncontrollably, which led to a rushed ER visit. Everyone assumed I was having a stroke or cardiac event. Then, after an hour or so, the symptoms stopped. Those assumptions were ruled out, yet no one knew what caused the episode.

I was fine from then until December, when I experienced all the same symptoms. I ended up in the ER twice, once even by ambulance. When everything was ruled out again, I was told to follow up with a cardiologist and neurologist. I did, and my cardiologist ran every test imaginable. All came back normal. My neurologist was convinced I had migraines presenting with "stroke-like symptoms." She put me on five different migraine medications and ran EEGs and CTs, all of which came back normal.

These episodes became more and more frequent. I'd experience a fast heart rate, low body temperature, low blood pressure, high blood pressure, brain fog, full body shakes, hand and arm tremors, twitches and tingling in my face, insomnia, focal aware seizures, double vision, headaches, chest pains, and severe anxiety. I quit going to the ER because they couldn't help me. I gave up on my cardiologist and neurologist, who seemed to do little more than offer guesses. I needed real help.

During one of my meltdowns, I had a moment of clarity: *I* was the only person who could offer me the help I needed, whether I felt like I was dying or not. I started documenting when the episodes occurred and noted what I was doing or eating beforehand. Through my system, I discovered that anything caffeinated and fermented triggered my episodes. When I eliminated all of those things, my episodes drastically reduced.

I was sure these were focal aware seizures, so I searched for neurologists who were likely to think outside of the box, really listen, and finally get me a diagnosis. My research led me to one, and I told her I had COVID in March 2020, confirmed by an antibody test, and that I didn't know whether it was related. She believed *all* of my symptoms directly resulted from my COVID infection. She believed that COVID-associated dysautonomia and POTS had damaged my nervous system. With the help of a cardiologist, new medication stabilized my blood pressure and body temperature. I had a glimmer of hope.

Then I started experiencing tremors in my hand, and my hopes were dashed. People were only just beginning to talk about Long COVID. Long haulers were experiencing extreme fatigue and breathing issues and about 50 other unexplained complications; they were finally talking about dysautonomia and seizures! I found a movement disorder specialist in New York, who discovered that my seizure medication was the likely culprit. My care team told me my nervous system needed more time to heal. They said it could take months, years, or, in the worst-case scenario, I might never fully recover. I wasn't ready to give up on my own research, though.

I discovered a treatment called Dynamic Neural Brain Retraining, recommended for people with extreme chemical sensitivities or, like me, with food triggers. I decided to give it a try, along with regular acupuncture treatments. By month six, I felt a massive difference in my body. One year into treatment, I was 85 percent better. I weaned off my anti-seizure medication and never had another. I reintroduced many foods and beverages to my diet with no relapsing symptoms. Some things could still trigger symptoms, but never anything as severe as a seizure.

I endured the lowest time in my life because of Long COVID. For me, this experience was worse than my cancer journey. Then, I at least had a concrete cancer diagnosis, a treatment plan, a dedicated health care team, and hope for full recovery. With COVID and Long COVID, I had absolutely none of that. For a long time, I wasn't sure whether I'd ever be able to talk about my near-complete recovery from COVID the way I could about cancer. Being on the front line of a growing medical question, alone with so much unknown, is a truly frightening place to be.

On the bright side, this brought me to the most brilliant and caring doctors. I bonded with dysautonomia and Long COVID patients and witnessed many of them reach the other side of their illness. Language emerged to describe our experiences. Long COVID clinics popped up nationwide, as did online support groups to help connect those in need.

I can tell you that it's pretty spectacular to be where I am now, knowing how far I've come to be able to look forward to a hopeful future. I am not the same person as I was before this began. This experience has changed me to my core, for better and worse. However, I make sure I focus on the good. While I work toward healing, I will continue to share my story. I never want anyone to experience the incredible difficulty that I did. If I can prevent that by sharing my story, I can give this nightmare a positive spin. Onward, upward and inward, every day.

To Whom It May Not Concern

Candis Freeman Johnson

ESSAY

To Whom It May Not Concern, if I could wish for one thing, it's that you understand the lasting effects of COVID-19. I'm a 40-year-old African American woman living a daily nightmare I cannot awaken from!

My entire family contracted COVID-19 during the first wave of the unknown virus in August 2020. Everyone recovered perfectly except me, thank God. I've had COVID-19 two more times since then, in January 2021 and October 2022, and I remain fully vaccinated. Most of the over a dozen doctors I saw did not believe my combination of bizarre symptoms. However, now I have a dedicated team of health care professionals who believe every word I say about my Long COVID diagnosis.

It wasn't always that way. I suffered for years of not being taken seriously by medical professionals who seemed so burned out, and not at all willing enough to go the extra mile needed to help me. Sometimes my blood work and CT scans would return normal. Yet I knew something was wrong because my symptoms never went away.

I spent a minimum of $3,000 a year, out of pocket, on exams my insurance wouldn't cover. I cried in doctors' offices when they couldn't answer me. I felt hopeless when yet another doctor would give me yet another referral to yet another specialist. Some weeks I was stuck in bed for days with excruciating pain throughout my body. I opened my eyes each morning and wondered, am I 40 or 99 years old? Every joint aches like I've just run a marathon I didn't train for.

My head pounds and my ears burn. All of my teeth hurt. My chest hurts. The constant tingling and burning in my legs is painful. I have no appetite but do have chills, night sweats, and a feverish feeling. Chronic fatigue weighs on me the most. I take three prescription meds in the morning and four at night, and several iron and immune support vitamins. When pain medication brings my pain scale from a 10 to a 5, I need an energy supplement boost to care for my children, spouse, animals, home, and self.

Before all of this, I was also the caregiver to my father-in-law, who has dementia. I cannot work full-time or even part-time since I have no clue how my body will feel from one day to the next. So I work flexible gigs that do not require a strict schedule: substitute teaching, Uber, and remote jobs. How can I care for my family without disability assistance due to significant restrictions? My accommodations are beyond reasonable at many companies. Neurological impairment sometimes makes it challenging to formulate a sentence, spell a word, or recall a memory, which also adds to the difficulty of gaining new employment. Long COVID left me with such a weak immune system. Imagine having the flu three or four times a week. I continue to wear a mask when I'm out of my home and around other people because I will always get sick. Trigeminal neuralgia creates the most excruciating pain flare-ups in my face, triggered by something as simple as chewing, applying makeup, or my body fighting more of this illness. Remaining in my bubble as much as possible to keep myself healthy is a slow process, but I am getting certified to become a beauty entrepreneur from home. I hope to generate income for my family like I did before COVID-19.

I've always been a homemaker, and my two daughters are my world. They depend on me in many ways. My parental duties used to include dropping them off and picking them up from school every day. They are now old enough to be self-sufficient in the mornings and take the bus to school. I'm no longer the mother I used to be and am always so fatigued, cranky from pain, emotional, and depressed from my bleak morning routine. However, I welcome them with hugs and kisses when they return home by 4:30. We eat dinner as a family with my wonderful partner, and I play like I'm back to being my normal self, refusing to focus on this nightmare. I just try to make the best of the few hours we have together before this nightmare begins all over again for me with each new day.

Before I had Long COVID, I loved traveling, baking desserts, thrift shopping, playing matchmaker to all my friends, feeding ducks with my girls, researching fashion, and just being creative and active. Today, most of my days are spent in bed trying to feel better. I still haven't adjusted to wearing hearing aids due to my Long COVID hearing impairment. For now, everyone who loves me will just have to continue to speak louder or repeat what they said, lol! As a natural optimist, I so LIVE for my good days and take many photos to capture those moments. Sometimes I'll share these photos with my support groups to help someone else who may be suffering while trying to get through a tough day.

Although Covid-19 infections have "gone away," according to many in the media, people like me still exist! We offer inputs for studies and clinical trials, all the while praying it leads to answers so that we can have a better quality of life. God is good!

Ice and the Pandemic

Rachel Baum

Here is where it flies and dies and rises
A warm sizzling slash across your back
The place where
Before the pandemic
A friend would briefly rest a palm.

No one ever said a walk in the woods would be
Innocent and vulnerable as the dog in his tweed coat.
He pauses near patches of exposed dirt to sense carrion in the air
Touches his nose to a jeaned leg—
This walk, after all, is for his benefit.

So despite the rip of razor wires
The quiet mean heat of constriction around your chest
You plod on
Eyeing warily the snow spattered ground
Knowing that ice lies beneath.

My Long COVID Storm

Patricia Milano

ESSAY

I am a 59-year-old veteran from Boston. I didn't think I would make it through the last three years as a COVID-19 survivor and long hauler.

Because of COVID-19, I lost all my personal belongings, a place to live, and almost my life and doggy, a 16-year-old Maltipoo named Zoro. I couldn't walk much or do any of my everyday routines. I spent thousands of dollars on over-the-counter products such as cough meds, Tylenol, Motrin, vitamins, minerals, creams, and lotions. None worked. I stayed with my son in Los Angeles for the second year and have been in a Boston veteran's homeless shelter for over seven months.

My COVID-19 began when I couldn't lift my head off the pillow one morning, and my body was stiff. It felt like I had pebbles going down my ear canals and inside my nostrils. My throat was on fire, and I had trouble swallowing; it felt like the inside of my mouth was full of sharp glass. My eyes were bleeding, and my brain felt like it was being squeezed by a vice grip. My hearing was impaired, and I had trouble speaking. I vomited and had diarrhea for days. I couldn't smell or taste anything and lost 40 pounds.

When I went into the hospital, the ambulance EMT told me that my left main heart ventricle was abnormal. He said my blood pressure was 190/40. I had small white grain-type bumps all over my face and body. Later, those turned to orange flame-type welts and hives all over my body. My skin was raised and burning for a year and a half, my hair fell in clumps, and I had trouble speaking. Black stuff came out of my nose. I coughed for almost two and a half years. I still have hot and cold electrical feelings from my toes to the top of my spine, and my whole body vibrates. I have trouble using my hands and fingers. I smell horrible trash-like things everywhere.

For the first time in our 13 years of togetherness, I had to find someone to care for Zoro. Zoro is in foster care with a great agency that will reunite us soon.

I am still struggling, but, despite everything, I feel very grateful to be alive.

Thor's Hammer

Abigail Koppes

ESSAY

One night, after almost passing out in the shower, I asked my husband to check my scalp. It felt like a thousand fire ants had burrowed into my skin. *Are there bugs inside of me?* It looked normal, so I thought it literally was in my head. That's what the doctors had said in the emergency room a few weeks earlier, but there was no way this was normal. I laid in bed trying not to move, but not sleeping, because the slightest shuffle was unbearable. Searing electric knives, or sometimes axes (take your pick), would select a random location to dig into my skull. It was like Thor's Hammer, shooting lightning behind the eyes. Sprinkle in some shortness of breath, dizziness, nausea, and blurry vision, but I thought the pain would surely kill me. A few days later, Thor returned and brought with him a soaring heart rate. Back to the emergency room I went. This time, the attending gave me a Xanax and, with IV fluids, said I was cleared to go home.

I started visualizing taking a fork in my kitchen and ripping the nerves out of the back of my head. That would fix it, right? It had to make the pain stop. Maybe they would believe me then. My eyes would blur and floating shapes would cross my vision and leave me breathless. The pang of the Hammer was never-ending. Three hours of sleep was a good night for me. I went on as a ghost of myself.

Five months later, my emergency consult got me into a neurology exam. The doctor suspected "typical" migraine, whatever that meant. Regardless of the swimming visions and flashing lights I saw, my eyes appeared normal. He took my history, hit my knees, listened to my story of eternal burning and stabbing. He diagnosed me, with kind regards, with migraine with aura. Then the medication roulette began.

My insurance mandated three front-line medications before I could get the good stuff; the meds that work better but cost more. All I had to show for five months of trials was failure, an allergic reaction to topiramate, some rashes, and shortness of breath. At this point (trigger warning), I thought about throwing myself in front of an oncoming commuter train or swimming out into the cold sea alone to make the pain *just stop.* Everyone except my husband said I looked fine. Invisible illness is like that. I slept two or four hours a night for eight months, regularly hallucinating. I often asked my husband if I was alive or dying. I cannot describe my deep despair for that man and our lost life together.

My attacks let up slowly, but daily symptoms remained. With a new injectable that cost about the same as rent, my migraines went from daily to a few per week. I still saw flashing lights, still couldn't sleep, still struggled for balance. I knew Thor's Hammer was lurking. At the grocery store one day, I dropped to the floor because of the pain in my left eye socket. That's a new fun spot, I thought as I gathered my food to check out. The ability to turn my head left or right was now gone, the muscles so tight that the skin on my skull started pulling down the back of my neck like a papier-mâché balloon. My hair fell out. I found no urgency with doctors, but they didn't know. Maybe it is stress. They often asked me if I was stressed.

Next stop was a pain clinic, where my neurologist suspected occipital neuralgia. Trauma or nerve impingement can cause Thor's burning and stabbing sensation in the back of the head. So, I received 30 lidocaine injections in my face, jaw, skull, neck, and shoulders; the pain was nothing compared to the Hammer, or an IUD insertion or broken bone. I felt numb, as expected, which was a positive diagnosis for occipital neuralgia. I was ecstatic for the 10 minutes it took to walk to the subway. I got on my train, it hit a bump, and pain zapped through my face. At least I had 10 minutes of peace.

My friends started disappearing. For them, I was out of sight and out of mind. I was working out of necessity but was a shell of myself. Talking hurt my face. Luckily my boss was understanding, and we worked out a way for me to be at home most of the time. A few excellent people stuck around to check on me, even against my will. My husband, the saint, held steady. It took six months to see any improvement in my pain with a cocktail of medications, regular acupuncture, massages, salt baths, and restrictive FODMAP diet. Yes, I was drinking enough water, thank you for asking.

My neurologist added more shots to my face and neck. He suspected trigeminal neuralgia and he was right. We found the Hammer. One fine day in June, I felt I "woke up" for the first time in a year. No one warns you that if you get COVID, as I did early into March's lockdown, neuralgia can pop into your life. I learned that trigeminal neuralgia is nicknamed the "Suicide Disease" and is quantifiably one of the most painful conditions known to (wo)man. There was no cure, but injections, physical therapy, and dietary changes could help alleviate symptoms. I was going about my daily life in more pain than giving birth or passing a kidney stone. What your body can stand is amazingly terrible. My pain team then referred me to rheumatology due to my swollen hands, white Raynaud's fingers, and a constellation of symptoms not expected with neuralgia. It turned out that I had new-onset Sjogren's Syndrome, an autoimmune disorder that often presents with neurological manifestations.

Did you know that your corneas need to be lubricated? I can't produce any tears, so crying was now a legitimate medical question. Two more meds were added. My remaining constellation of symptoms, my stars in the sky, were also beyond Sjogren's, so autonomic testing was next. I figured a tilt-table test will be as routine as anything. My heart rate sometimes skyrocketed unexpectedly, and stairs were difficult, but I could stand for short periods. They took a chunk of skin from my ankle to check for a kind of nerve death called small fiber neuropathy. That would explain the fire ants and the tingling in my fingers and toes all day and night. The tilt throws me for a loop, like my stomach fell out on the floor in front of the technician's Keds. I told him I'm going to vomit, but he was nonplused. I was diagnosed with postural orthostatic tachycardia syndrome (POTS). Oh good, now even gravity was against me. My autonomic nervous system was haywire, which brought more medications to counteract my overactive fight-or-flight response.

POTS is frequently misdiagnosed as anxiety, especially for women. Might I also be hysterical, they asked me. I told them I think I'm pretty hysterical(ly funny). Off-label Mestinon did its job of allowing my parasympathetic nervous system to appropriately tighten the blood vessels in my legs when I stood. Suddenly, I had fewer heart rate episodes and could function for a couple of hours a day before crashing.

Thor's Hammer still reared its head and knocked me flat, especially if I got dehydrated or moved my head too quickly. POTS kept blood and oxygen from my muscles and brain, and my muscles and brain needed blood and oxygen to function. That explained a lot. My new normal was eating five to eight grams of sodium, drinking liters of water, and living in compression gear to funnel that blood north. Over the coming months, the muscles in my neck let their guard down bit by bit, and baby hairs appeared out of nowhere as blood replenished my dying scalp.

After two years, I can do a few hours of work daily and see my friends or family every week or so. The Hammer is now the size of one of those tiny tool kits you have in your dorm room in college. It's still big enough to do damage, but it visits less frequently. Thor and I are learning to live together (me more than him). For this, there is no cure. I teach and have been able to be on my feet enough to do my job with modifications. I now mentor my students virtually, though both they and I know it's not the same. I have to lie down afterward, dead to the world, but at least I get a glimpse of "the before times" through my screen. I love my job and grieve for it often. I can sleep a little better now. *I can write this.*

I'll continue to biohack: Doctors don't have all the answers here. Long COVID is new, and many are still dismissive of its existence. I host my own GNC inside my medication cabinet, built on the research of strangers on the internet and the brave doctors willing to stand for us. I give them what I can: stellate ganglion blocks, MRIs, PET scans, nattokinase, my blood, my labs. Take these and use them for those after me, I hope.

I dream about running, skiing, laughing, and walking my dogs. I have nightmares about who, if anyone, will believe us? Will I have children? Is help coming? I think those answers must be written in Thor's constellations.

The Longest Part of Long Covid

Tim Murphy

Maybe there's no distinction
between invisible
and visible illnesses.
Maybe we simply choose
which ones to see.
Like how we avert our gaze

from millions of people sick
with a virus we cannot see
but know follows us,
spread so casually
one could almost mistake
all of this as inevitable.

Because the longest part of Long Covid,
of being disabled in a pandemic
rendered endless
by declaring over too soon,
isn't this merciless illness,
nor anyone of its many symptoms,

it's that I'll never unsee this mass forgetting,
how quickly, quietly the convenience of
friends, family, strangers usurped
the safety and inclusion of sick people like me,
who lack the luxury of breathing this air
we share when masks no longer scrub it.

And so I stand in line at the grocery store,
and I tremble,
as I look into a sea
of naked faces and see
staring back at me expired empathy, mass apathy,
and I feel, I feel closing in around me,

the confines of this small world we've built,
where it's easier to endanger than to feel,
safer to harm than to heal,
and I think to myself,
until I can think of nothing else,
that I am most lonely in a room full of people.

What a Virus Awoke in Me

Tim Murphy

Days enmesh,
their only common thread
a fog pierced only by dread
that this long,
cyclic sickness
will know no end.

I read but words dance,
strike concussive blows I've known,
but this time, without touching me.
Music, once a respite, now a trigger
pulled by the robin's high note I hear
singing, ringing in my ear,

every sound too loud,
every light too bright,
walking my dogs,
high stakes roulette,
a block too far,
and I am punctured

by this ever-looming crash
and its too-sharp teeth
that scar deeper than skin,
as the room now swims,
my body bobs, sways,
lurches, until I am lying, vacant,

on the cold titled floor, unable to move,
nor remove the word *help*
from behind frozen lips,
my mind, dazed, splintered, ruptured
like it was in the moments
just after impact of those volcanic concussions

I hoped, I begged, I thought long extinct
but merely lay dormant,
now awoken, rumbling,
erupting anew,
now unleashed by this virus that will not sleep,
now relived inside me each long waking day.

A Walking Meditation on Long COVID

Judith Rosenbaum

ESSAY

I breathe in slowly and let it out, focusing on the expansion of my lungs, the feel of the cold air as it passes through my nostrils, and the warm air out through my throat. I am learning to meditate. My face itches, my mind jumps frenetically; I feel my irregular heartbeat pounding in my chest. I focus on my breath and yawn repeatedly as if, in paying attention to my breath, my body has forgotten how to breathe. I find it hard to sit still, to commit time to doing what seems to be nothing.

It's been two and a half years since I contracted COVID-19 (in August 2020), and I am still struggling with its symptoms. My body aches, my joints wince and weird electrical currents buzz at my skin and the top of my skull. My brain is shrouded in a fog that no amount of coffee can clear; words slip behind an impenetrable wall; my heart slows way down and then suddenly speeds up, beating irregularly; my feet are simultaneously numb and painful. These strange symptoms wax and wane, and while not severe enough to keep me from functioning altogether, it is obvious to me and those closest to me that I'm functioning at reduced capacity. ("Sure, you've had some cognitive decline," my husband observes, quickly reassuring me, "but don't worry — you at 80 percent is as good as anyone else at 100 percent!" I am not reassured.) I can't quite remember what normal felt like, but I know this isn't it.

It's the uncertainty that gets me. Waking, I reach tentatively into my limbs to take stock. Will this be a good day or a bad day? Before I've even fully awakened, before I've stood up and let the blood flow through my limbs, I can feel the weight of each cell, an uncomfortable reverberation, a cloudy veil over my mind. Not a good day.

I need rest, but it was never modeled for me. My mom, despite several recurrences of cancer, was always doing. Not in the active, athletic sense — she didn't run or play tennis or climb mountains, or even walk particularly fast. (She always stopped if she had something important to say, which was often. This made her an emphatic but irritating walking companion.) She could sit on the couch for hours, but always with something to read: a crossword or a deck of cards. Stillness was not her thing.

Now, I am trying to learn to tune in to my body, which takes effort since I was not encouraged to cultivate it as a skill. As a runner on the high school cross country and track teams, I was taught to push through the pain, not let it guide me. As a daughter, too, I internalized the message to disregard the limitations of the body and keep going, one foot in front of the other. My mother did so, barely pausing, even when recuperating from surgery, chemo, or radiation.

One foot in front of the other. This is the tradition of resilience in which I was raised. Push through the pain, keep your eyes trained on what you're trying to achieve. Keep moving. Don't stop, don't rest. A tradition of ambition, of urgency, of bravery, perhaps. Of transcending the limits of the body.

I suspect this is a deeply rooted inheritance from generations of Jewish refugees who had to keep moving to stay alive. My existence makes the case for its effectiveness. And this approach served my mother well, too. Stage 4 cancer barely slowed her down. Despite decades of surgeries, chemo, and radiation, she wrote, taught, pioneered a new field of study, and pursued new challenges and goals.

Who am I, then, to pause? Who am I to lie down merely because my clothes feel leaden, to curl into my aching body? It feels unnatural. My instinct is to push.

Long COVID demands that I reframe my approach to living. For months, I kept pushing, denying my symptoms, assuming that I'd eventually build back my strength and feel normal again, and in the meantime, I just had to keep moving forward. Fake it till you make it, medical edition. The fundamental lesson of Long COVID — I am still learning — is to rest, listen to my body, and not push it. Exertion triggers Long COVID symptoms, so I must tune in so deeply that I learn what will sap my strength before I start to feel it. Recovery is always two steps forward, one step back. I must stop expecting a linear path to healing.

As I drag myself through my days, limbs aching and heavy with exhaustion, I feel compassion for my mother, who must have tuned out so much pain to get through her years of treatment and recovery. As a child, I turned away from any reminders of her illness, as if that could make her healthy and normal.

And frankly, I also feel angry. Angry that I wasn't taught to develop the skills of listening to my body. Angry that developing my mind was always the priority, at the expense of investing in respect for the needs and limits of my body. It is hard to rewire in midlife.

Deep breath in, slow release. Return the mind to the breath. Again and again. Notice what I'm feeling and keep breathing. My foot falls asleep, and I shift slightly. "One foot in front of the other." Sometimes it's my mother's voice I hear. Sometimes it's my grandmother, a fierce, stubborn, and energetic matriarch in her own right, who for 94 years overcame many hardships and obstacles — poverty, motherlessness, abuse — through sheer force of will. How will I unlearn the instinct to push myself and keep marching on? How will I learn to pause and be in the moment, especially when doing so feels like a repudiation of my maternal lineage?

"One foot in front of the other" is a command to keep marching when doing so feels impossible. But now its echo suggests a different, more mindful meaning. Perhaps there's an element of presence in "one foot in front of the other." At least there's an acknowledgment that you can only take one step at a time. One breath and then another. That's how we live — noticing that process by focusing on the breath. Tentatively, I transform the directive "one foot in front of the other" from a forced march into a walking meditation. Before COVID-19 made it impossible, I was a runner, pounding out anxiety with each stride. Now, I've changed my pace. In my mind's eye, I am in the woods, taking slow, intentional steps, placing my foot down firmly, and moving forward differently. Not running, no longer pushing my body to obey my will, but instead harnessing the discipline to slow the daily march to one step, one breath, at a time. A march no longer; it is now a meditative dance; two steps forward, one step back.

The Journey to the Bench

Rowan MacDonald

ESSAY

I don't leave home without it: the blue backpack that contains my survival kit. Pills to slow a racing heart, breath mints to calm a dry mouth, travel sickness tablets for nausea. I'm not joining a vessel in rough seas or flying by plane; I'm simply leaving the house, attempting a task many take for granted. The wallet and library card in my jeans pocket are optimistic at best, remnants of previous abilities. I won't reach the library or the shopping center. To leave the house, though, and put one foot in front of the other is to stand in defiance. *Might as well go down swinging, I guess.*

Approaching the neighbor's fence causes me to search the bottom of my backpack for a get-out-of-jail-free card: my iPod. Pausing too long risks losing the afternoon, momentum, and sanity. There's movement in the window and a curtain flaps. *Shit.* My elderly neighbor, Mavis, loves to chat. She's an independent 87-year-old with more stamina and strength than me, a 32-year-old man. Society expects me to protect the vulnerable, to shield the likes of Mavis from those in society wishing to cause harm, to assist wherever possible. Society doesn't expect an afternoon chat with her to leave me weakened, lightheaded, and forced to abort a short walk. So, conversations with Mavis take place over the fence instead.

This journey requires steely determination, because my symptoms grow with each step, occasionally rising to the surface. Such symptoms need chess-game concentration levels to push through. Once I escape Mavis, I shuffle through my iPod, searching for the right track to propel me up the hill ahead. My playlist is quintessentially '90s and brims with nostalgia. It reflects a man who's checked out of 2023, chosen to live in a simpler era when life was happier. I pause and look up at the incline, my intense focus no different now than in the 100-meter blocks when I was a sprinter, back when I was healthy. Back to another life entirely.

Despite possessing the name Redwood Road, there aren't any redwoods in sight. The only trees are old maples, swaying in the breeze beside a nursing home. On a good day, I pass the mailbox at number 28 before gasping for air. I'm going to require a pit stop once I reach the entrance to the nursing home. It's the same one where my grandmother took her last breath. I hover awkwardly on the sidewalk, sucking in oxygen and feigning interest in my phone. I pretend to look for directions to hide the fact I'm spent after walking just 800 feet. An older man pushes a walking frame on the opposite side of the road. He shuffles with confident perseverance before stopping to check for traffic. He's not out of breath.

Step by step, I pass a vandalized mailbox that sends my letters to overseas pen pals. These kinds of low-maintenance friendships don't require me to meet anyone at scheduled times or abruptly cancel plans. It's a social life via airmail, like traveling without leaving the couch. Whenever I drop letters in the box, I ponder the vast distances these envelopes will travel and how they're so much farther than anything I'm capable of.

I feel good today, so I attempt the roundabout. It's not much farther, but the steep rise makes me feel like I'm climbing a mountain. At the top, it would be tempting to radio base camp to beg Sherpas for oxygen, but there is no assistance and no oxygen here. It's just me, my two jelly legs, and the route home. I gulp from my water bottle and pretend to look for directions again. Anything to prevent society from knowing this young man is exhausted from the shortest of walks up the smallest of hills. I'm paranoid that someone might ask if I'm lost, so I start back down. Google tells me the distance is a measly 500 yards.

I never venture past the roundabout. Life descends into anarchy past the roundabout. People get stabbed past the roundabout. I'm dealing with enough pain and discomfort without adding a stab wound to the mix. My slow walk is already accompanied by traffic noise that assaults my senses and overwhelms me. Reprieve is found in the little alleyway that travels between houses. The array of bird calls provides a welcome distraction from the graffiti-littered fence. A black crow struts up and down the telephone wire overhead, squawking for comrades to join him in afternoon high jinks. Occasionally, when the ocean swells pick up, seagulls try their luck at taking over the crows' wire.

The local nursing home is a godsend, because it's responsible for the row of benches lining the path to the supermarket. The benches make life easier for the elderly residents, and for someone like me. I use these benches every day. If I'm feeling particularly adventurous, I may only use one or two. I never actually know how far I can walk, but my goal is always the bench that overlooks the Barn, our local market. It's where I catch my breath and gaze up at clouds rolling over the snowcapped mountains in the distance. It's where I wonder if a "normal" body will return to me someday. That bench is where I mourn my pre-COVID life. Today, I'm going to make it. *Knees start to buckle, strides quicken, vision blurs.*

I slump onto the red wood with my backpack in my lap. An afternoon breeze whistles through the tall, unkempt grass around me. Bursts of sunlight bounce off car windshields in the parking lot below. A blue jay pecks at a pine cone in a tall pine tree. I close my eyes and ignore the cigarette butts and broken beer bottles at my feet. I meditate. I breathe. I give thanks for being able to summit this Everest today, for reaching a graffiti-ridden bench and cigarette butts and broken glass. Because by making it here, I have overcome my broken body.

This daily journey is my last remaining connection to the world, since I rarely go anywhere else. But I can walk, so I do. I walk for my grandmother, who was in a wheelchair for 50 years. I walk for all those bedridden in hospitals and homes. I walk for myself, so I don't lose the ability. And I walk for the many millions like me battling ME/CFS and Long COVID.

My View from a Bench

Jennifer Kreatsoulas

ESSAY

On a sunny day in August 2022, I sat on a bench on the boardwalk in Ocean City, New Jersey, waiting for my husband and two young daughters to pass by on the bikes we rented for the morning. Bike rides on the boards after pancakes at Bob's Grill is one of our favorite vacation traditions. This was our first trip back to Ocean City since the pandemic hit.

While watching the sun's rays reflect off the ocean, I had a flashback: I was sitting on a bench just like this one, on this very boardwalk, many summers ago with my grandparents and sister, eating an orange-and-vanilla swirl cone from Kohr Brothers. When reminiscing about those carefree summers of jumping waves, playing paddleball on the beach, and going on the amusement rides after sunset, I didn't feel nostalgia. What I felt was the unrelenting sense of loss and grief, one that had increasingly permeated my being for the past three years. I was 44 when I became ill with COVID, and I've never gotten better.

My family would ride by any moment, and I was determined to give them an enthusiastic wave. Now was not the time to remember how much I loved riding a bike on the trails near our house, running in the quiet of early morning sunshine, rock climbing at the local gym, hiking with my family in autumn, or walking the dog through our neighborhood. Now was not the time for sorrow over how separate I feel from a world that moves so quickly or for giving in to the longing for my life before Long COVID. Now was not the time to be swept away by the trauma of not knowing if I or the tens of millions of people around the world who have been affected by this mass disabling event will ever recover our health.

Living with Long COVID means I have not been able to drive. Thirty minutes in the car as a passenger is my limit before some of my symptoms, particularly debilitating fatigue, body aches, and brain fog, escalate too much. Ocean City is about 90 minutes from home, so I knew this trip would take a toll before we even arrived. Still, I insisted we come. Life must go on, I told myself, for the people I love, if not for me.

I strained my brain to keep steady focus amid the hundreds of passersby on wheels or feet. The sound of the waves rolling, children's joyful laughter, seagulls calling, music streaming from various storefronts, challenged my cognition. This is the vibrant energy I have always loved to immerse myself in, but it felt as if my brain was short-circuiting from the stimulation. Whenever my nervous system becomes overloaded, I experience this sensation and an often-accompanying difficulty finding my words. I dared not think about the inevitable crash that would soon compromise my mobility and functioning even more than usual. And when the oncoming crash did cross my mind, I bargained with myself that at least I'd be nonfunctional at the beach rather than on the couch at home. Even that couldn't console me about all that I was missing out on.

The balance between crashing and participating in life seems to be unavoidable with this illness. Now, leaving the house is dependent on how far the drive is, how far the walk is, and where I can sit down midway. In the first year of this illness, I'd often try to walk in the driveway or in front of our house. I walked so slowly that the neighbors worried that I had had a stroke or speculated that I was recovering from a hip replacement. It was just too embarrassing to acknowledge how I moved was being perceived by others, so I started walking in the backyard instead. Three years into living with Long COVID, my capacity is still only a few laps around the yard.

Perhaps my husband and mother had been right that a wheelchair would have helped me to conserve energy and do more on our three-day trip, but the reality the chair represented was too devastating to accept, too traumatic. I chose the bench, which was hard enough to accept. For good or bad, I still choose to rely on my own two legs. This illness has demanded that I give up so much already. Holding on to my mobility, to personal agency, may impact my physical health at times, but I am acutely aware of how doing so is keeping my emotional and mental health afloat. Eventually, I'll need to make peace with a wheelchair, but not now. No matter how debilitated I'd be by the end of this trip, I assured myself it was worth it because I would gain the peace of mind that we gave our girls a vacation, my husband would have joy in his life, we were still making memories together, and my family's life could continue even if mine was nearly at a standstill.

After resting slumped on the bench for several minutes, I repositioned myself to sit tall and upright and appear alert in time for my family to pass by. Choosing my battles in moments like this one keeps me engaged and surviving the physical and mental challenges of Long COVID. Depression and anxiety are also symptoms of this illness. Washing dishes, making my bed, packing my daughters' lunches, feeding the dog: Mundane tasks help me feel connected to my life. The flip side, however, is that the exertion that engaging requires adds up quickly, and it's only a matter of time until my symptoms intensify. Experts call this the push-crash or boom-bust cycle. I still haven't found my way out of it, mostly because I am a parent raising a young family and, in truth, these tasks feel like a lifeline. They carry me through days that feel heavy and endless when you are housebound and need to rely on others to take you to the bank or the coffee shop. I've found lifelines in warm tea, cozy socks, snuggles with my girls, poetry, calls with friends, the *Harry Potter* movies, nature documentaries, my red heated blanket, sitting in the sun, my dog, therapy, and connecting with others affected by Long COVID.

I wrote my second book, *The Courageous Path to Healing*, before getting COVID. It shares my story of eating disorder recovery and, through reflection exercises inspired by my work as a certified yoga therapist, invites readers to recognize their own courage. It's not lost on me that now, once again, I am required to be courageous. Not until living with a chronic illness like Long COVID did I understand how isolating it can be, and how much it can shrink a once-expansive life. I haven't figured out how to fully accept my new reality and make the hope for healthier days easier to access. The best I can do is approach the concept of moving forward as a daily practice, which takes the form of choosing to get out of bed, getting dressed, eating meals with my family, keeping in contact with my friends, and making responsible choices for my physical and mental health. It often means maintaining a routine, accommodating my capacity on any given day, and saying no to most social activities and long car rides.

I knew the trip to Ocean City was far beyond my capacity. Feeling the ocean breeze against my back, I remembered my therapist saying that my presence matters more to my family than how much or how little I can do. Although I wasn't on a bike, they knew I was with them, that I was present on the bench. This was the bittersweet comfort I needed most: They knew I was still showing up. Their mother and wife, while changed by illness, was committed to being present for them every day. And for that reason alone, I will sit on as many benches as I have to throughout my life.

I spotted my husband's smile and heard my daughters' laughter. I perked up and cheered as I waved to them. They waved back and blew me kisses, full of joy to be in a place they love. And as quickly as the sun was on their faces heading toward me, it was on their backs as they sped away. I watched from my bench and awaited their return.

Acceptance and Gratitude with Long COVID

John Zeising

Everything I go through,
I get through, I grow through.
Everything that exits my life is
always replaced by something even
better. I never lack.
— @WeTheUrban on Twitter, March 30, 2023

The best way to find yourself is to lose yourself in the service of others.
— Mahatma Gandhi

ESSAY

My name is John, but when I was a firefighter, everyone knew me as "Z." Originally from New York, I live in the mountains of Colorado with my partner. For the last 24 of my 31 years in Colorado, I have been in the fire service, initially as a volunteer and then as a paid career structural firefighter and paramedic.

I have always been active and fit, playing hockey, running marathons, hiking and climbing 14,000 foot peaks, and bike riding across this amazing state. Now I am disabled by Long COVID.

A good day for me is having enough energy, with my pain and other symptoms under control, to go to the grocery store or maybe see live music in our small town for an hour before my battery is drained. On a bad day, I am laid up in bed with neuropathy flaring in my feet and legs, fatigue so heavy it feels like gravity has doubled, my heart beating erratically despite the installation of a pacemaker post-COVID, my skull feeling like it is being split open by an ax, my thoughts and speech slow and slurred, and an electrical-like constant buzzing in my head that the doctors call tinnitus. When I get up, I use a walker, as my dysautonomia and POTS can suddenly bring on a near syncopal (fainting or passing out) episode.

Fortunately, more than two years after my initial infection in December 2020, my good days have become more frequent, and my worst symptom flares are less severe. Monthly immunoglobulin infusions are tamping down my neurological symptoms from the small nerve fiber neuropathy.

However, from a physical activity standpoint, I am a shadow of who I was before. If I exert myself too much physically, mentally, or emotionally, my symptoms come roaring back, landing me in bed. This phenomenon is known as PEM, or Post Exertional Malaise. To me, "malaise" is an understatement.

Approximately 10 million people here in the United States, and upward of 60 million more worldwide, have never fully recovered from their COVID-19 infections. And even though the daily infection and death rates have dropped dramatically from the highs of 2021, in winter 2023 there were still more than 300 Americans dying daily from the virus. And untold numbers of those who survive will eventually join the Long COVID club.

To date, researchers have not definitively determined why some of us have not recovered from COVID-19. Thus a cure, rather than just therapies, has yet to be found. Over 200 potential signs and symptoms are associated with Long COVID, many of which overlap with or are similar to other syndromes like Lyme disease, post-MERS, and myalgic encephalomyelitis/ chronic fatigue syndrome (ME/CFS).

Unfortunately, since the start of the pandemic too many medical professionals have been circumspect about the failure of some COVID patients to recover, with some even advocating just "pushing through," getting fresh air, and exercising. This "treatment" has caused patients who took the advice to experience repeated flare-ups of our worst symptoms.

Other medical professionals have straight up gaslit many of us and referred us to mental health professionals with the unsaid (or stated) presumption that our physical symptoms are manifestations of depression or anxiety.

I struggle with depression. However, I think it is warranted. First, I lost my health, and I have no idea if and when I'll ever return to an age-appropriate health level again. I feel like I have aged 20 years in the two and a half years since I became sick.

Second, I lost a career that I loved. Being a firefighter/paramedic is a job that beats up the body, mind, and soul, but it also provided great purpose and meaning in my life.

Third, I can now do only a few activities and hobbies I love aside from work, whether running or hiking, climbing a mountain, traveling for pleasure or medical missions, attending social activities, or practicing photography, which has been a lifelong passion.

Fourth, my illness has brought economic fears. While I am fortunate that I applied for and received disability from my firefighters' pension association, my take-home pay is less than it was. And on top of that, I have lost out on future earnings and raises, along with contributions to my retirement accounts, and now have to pay for my private health insurance.

Under COBRA laws, I have access to health insurance from my employer for three years, and then I will have to shop for a new policy, which will be very expensive due to my medical history. I will be too young to access Medicare and unable to apply for Social Security Disability Income because career firefighters covered by a pension don't contribute to Social Security. Thus, we are not eligible for benefits, even if we worked for years in the private sector before becoming firefighters.

All that said, as I have trudged my way through numerous medical appointments and procedures over the past 27 months, I have not only slowly gained acceptance for my condition, but I have also found gratitude. The acceptance isn't to say I'm just lying down and resigning myself to my new reality. No. While continuing to seek out therapies that help, I accept that this is just a new challenge presented to me in this life, and there is much I can learn from it.

That means having greater empathy for others with chronic illnesses or disabilities, especially those like Long COVID that do not come with visible signs. Invisibility is accompanied by the hardship of not being believed or accepted by others. When I pull into an accessible parking space and hang my handicapped placard, I get dirty or disapproving looks from passersby if I walk under my own power into the grocery store, feeling well enough not to use my walker.

I have found gratitude over the small things that I never used to notice.

I pay closer attention now, whether to a sunrise or sunset, the efforts by my partner to help make me comfortable or watch for signs that I might be flaring, or family and friends that stay in touch and visit to help or bring meals.

And beyond, or possibly intertwined with, acceptance and gratitude, is a slowly developing and evolving mission to find purpose and meaning each day. It may not be the type I felt and received in my career, but it is still to be striven for. Whether that is helping my partner in some small way to express my appreciation for her, calling a friend who is struggling with illness or injury, participating in Long COVID support groups, helping with political action for chronic illness patients, or even writing and sharing as I am doing here in the hope that it will help someone else as much as it helps me.

And it means holding the dream of one day being able to do many of the things I used to enjoy. Even if those goals are not attainable, I appreciate the knowledge I have gained and now have a new and different community full of positive and inspiring people.

This isn't the journey I planned on. But sometimes, the best adventures are ones not of our own design.

Living with Chronic Lymphocytic Leukemia and COVID-19

David Charles Braun

In 2016, I was diagnosed with chronic lymphocytic leukemia, which the American Cancer Society defines as a type of cancer that develops from your white blood cells, the lymphocytes in your bone marrow. When COVID-19 arrived in the U.S., I began safeguarding myself and stopped attending large gatherings, which made sense because my immune system remained compromised by my leukemia. But, like all those who were essential personnel, I was never given the opportunity to work from home. I continued going in everyday, the risk becoming my new normal.

ESSAY

Before Jan. 17, 2022, I was an avid outdoorsman busy with many hobbies: I conducted studies of bald eagles as a naturalist and volunteered for the Department of Natural Resources, I fished, went camping, and often was birding. Then COVID-19 changed everything. On Jan. 17, 2022, I was admitted to the emergency room by ambulance. A doctor stood over me while I lay on the gurney and asked if I had ever been trached, intubated, ventilated, or had any last rites. I spent two weeks there with internal bleeding requiring blood transfusions, COVID-19, COVID pneumonia, A-Fib ...

I was then moved to recovery. I was unable to walk and take care of myself. Nurses would clean, bathe, and ask me to roll left and right to change my bedding. I spent the next six weeks between two rehab facilities where I learned how to walk again, always fighting fatigue and shortness of breath. I returned home in March and continued home health care and therapy.

I lost my job of 22 years due to COVID-19. I quickly used all of my PTO and short-term disability. I filed for disability and unemployment benefits at the suggestion of my lawyer, along with a forbearance with my mortgage lender for six months. I couldn't find work. As the primary breadwinner in my family, I knew my unemployment assistance would soon expire. My wife continued to work grueling hours for FedEx, but my health took a toll on all of us. She gave up countless nights of sleep, driving the slick winter roads between me at the hospital, her days at work, and the difficult task of managing our home alone; I'm very grateful to her. In December 2022, we were blessed with my disability coverage. Soon after, we sold our family house and moved outside of Indianapolis.

As a long hauler, I still use a walker and experience fatigue and shortness of breath. I can't say I feel like my old self, but my relationship with God is more potent: I feel less like I take my life for granted now, and I have a greater clarity since COVID-19 that I, along with my wife and older brother, am here to care for my 91-year-old mother and hold close the memory of my brother Dan, whom I recently lost. I often feel like the eagles I used to watch so dearly: They've made their way back from near-extinction after catastrophic destruction and danger. I look at them, with their resilience and adaptability, and think maybe I can, too. I hope to be reunited with them someday.

Long COVID

Cynthia Read Gardner

In company
I pretend to taste
gamble on knowing
what I need

discard
what may be spoiled
having lost the sense
to smell danger

working through
certainty
with no compulsion
for evidence

what's left is
the idea
of taste
texture of sustenance
like the grip

I remember
as your arm
around my waist
like the newly blind remember
frozen in time
the essence of face

Gone but Never Forgotten

Haley Nelson

ESSAY

I know what it's like to disappear.

I know what it's like to be confined to 14 by 16 feet for 22 hours of the day, suffocated by medical equipment, fluorescent orange pill bottles, tennis trophies, academic awards, and Polaroid pictures of the girl I once knew.

To have friends and family fabricate their conclusions about your illness:

She just needs to try a little harder; this does not happen to healthy young people.

I had the flu before and was really sick for like two weeks, so I know exactly how she feels.

Probably psychiatric problems ... very popular with young ladies, you know.

To encounter doctors who don't take you seriously and give you false hope of a speedy recovery:

Well, you weren't hospitalized with COVID, so it really shouldn't be this severe.

POTS? Could be. Can you resend that research study? Must've misplaced it in my inbox.

Conversion disorder: your physical symptoms are a result of repressed trauma.

I know what it's like to watch the world from your window. It goes on without you as days melt into weeks, weeks into months, months into one year, eight months, and six days. But who's counting?

I also know this: I refuse to be lost forever.

Let's start from the beginning.

Hi, my name is Haley and I am 19 years old. I am a world traveler, self-proclaimed U.S. history geek, avocado-toast enthusiast, iced coffee connoisseur, and *Dateline* fanatic. My favorite color is seafoam green because it reminds me of summers spent sea-glass hunting at the Jersey Shore. I am described by those who know me best as a hard worker, perfectionist, and serial smiler.

The story (turned nightmare) begins in June 2021, at the end of my junior year. A month I will never forget.

It started like every teenage coming-of-age film: chaos as final assessments busied the last week of school, gossip as last-minute after-prom plans flooded group chats, and collective anxiety and excitement as we tweaked our Common App essays and manifested acceptances into top universities. My biggest concerns were presenting my prototype for an engineering final and finding the perfect high heels to match my prom dress.

Life was as it was meant to be, until it wasn't.

I remember the last good morning like it was yesterday.

Surrounded by evidence of s'mores from the night before, abandoned sparkly dresses and heels, and my six close girlfriends from high school, I woke up smiling. After prom had been a success.

Determined to make it to my 2 o'clock tennis clinic, I gathered my things, threw on my UCLA hoodie sporting last night's makeup, and drove home, stopping to pick up Dunkin'.

Only I never made it to my tennis clinic. With a raw throat, stuffy nose, and abnormally watery eyes that I could barely keep open, I decided I was over-exhausted from the night before. Confident that a few-hour nap was all I needed to revive myself, I crawled under the covers.

The next morning, I woke to the fluorescent glow of my phone. I opened Snapchats from "After Prom 2021" and quickly learned I was not the only one who caught what people were already calling "the prom plague." Empathizing with photos of NyQuil and homemade chicken soup sent by friends, I managed a laugh, which produced a sharp pain in my throat.

Days passed, or so I am told, as I soon fell into a comatose state and lost all concept of time, and I was the only one who did not improve.

"Isolate for two weeks and take vitamin D and zinc. You are young and healthy, Haley — you will be back to it in no time," I was assured.

My case of Covid-19 was what doctors called mild — a loss of smell and taste, headaches, and flu-like, gastrointestinal, and sinus symptoms that lasted for about two weeks. Yes, I was "young and healthy." But no, I was not "back to it in no time."

Post-infection, I experienced profound fatigue, intense brain fog and memory loss, headaches, and a feeling that something "just wasn't right." "Mild" was the understatement of the century.

I struggled to recall simple drills as a tennis instructor, felt like I had run a marathon after practices that used to feel easy to me, and had trouble finding the right words, organizing my thoughts, and following conversations. But I pushed through like I always did. My parents and I agreed that my lingering symptoms should subside in a few weeks. We were wrong.

Upon starting my senior year in September, my symptoms exacerbated and multiplied. Before, I was an Energizer bunny — I would attend school, head student council meetings, lead class discussions, meet with clubs, thrive at Varsity tennis practice and matches, and still have enough energy to tend to volunteer commitments, homework, and studying. My post-COVID routine was vastly different. My limbs felt so heavy that getting out of bed and leaving the house felt nearly impossible. My poor memory and concentration made me forget the route I had taken countless times before to school. Following class content required immense effort and energy; time on the tennis court led to dizziness and heart palpitations, which resulted in malaise so severe that I would collapse in bed afterward from exhaustion, and showering left my limbs purple, white, and numb.

"Hey, Haley, are you all right?" became as commonplace as "Hello."

After nearly collapsing one day that fall during a student council meeting, I could no longer ignore my body's pleas for help.

Unsure where to turn, a family friend suggested we meet with a neurologist who noted my motor function was fine and suggested my high heart rate and fatigue resulted from anxiety and stress about applying to colleges. I felt dismissed, disbelieved, and insulted. This individual could not have been more wrong.

While my parents and I figured out the next steps, I kept pushing through, and surprise — I kept getting worse. I could barely keep my eyes open during the day. I experienced a lead-like feeling in my limbs that craved inertia. Tingling. Numbness. Temperature dysregulation and digestion problems. Brain fog. Dizziness. An out-of-body sensation. Excruciating headaches. Newfound sensitivity to light and sound.

My symptoms grew so intense that attending high school virtually was my only option to graduate on time. It was a struggle. Cyclical flare-ups of exacerbated symptoms that left me bed-bound were preceded by swollen lymph nodes, a sore throat, and that lead-like limb feeling. It felt like my body was rebelling against me.

As my symptoms worsened, my family and I worked with various doctors who collectively diagnosed me with Post-acute Covid-19 Syndrome/Long COVID. With so little information and research, I felt like a guinea pig with physicians trying different medications to address each of my many symptoms. And somehow, the details of how I presented myself — whether or not I could manage to put on makeup that day, whether or not my parents helped me find the right words to explain how miserable I felt, and whether or not the tears I shed from the utter frustration and exhaustion of it all made me "an emotional liability" — were always relevant enough to include in after-visit notes.

Eventually, through connection with my visiting nurse, I met with two specialists who performed extensive testing and ordered enough blood work to make the Labcorp employees do triple takes.

Myalgic Encephalomyelitis/Chronic Fatigue Syndrome. Postural Orthostatic Tachycardia Syndrome (POTS). Small Fiber Neuropathy.

After receiving the news, I remember crying and then laughing. Was it an inappropriate response? A healthy person would likely say yes. But I can guarantee you that most patients would say it was perfectly appropriate.

I now had names for what early doctors made me believe "was all in my head." Names for what select friends and family members discounted. Names affirming the nightmare I was battling daily.

These names, yet oddly comforting, of course, do not provide resolve.

In sharing my experience, I acknowledge my privilege and recognize I am luckier than most regarding receiving support and care.

My parents have been my biggest advocates and believers since Day One. Support systems for many patients take a lot of work to come by.

Obtaining an accurate diagnosis is rare, and even then, often happens years later due to the roaring inequities that bind our health care system.

If you take one thing away from this essay, I hope it be this:

I am still missing.

Missing from the college classes I would have been taking.

Missing from the family gatherings I so desperately want to attend without ending up in bed, comatose from fatigue.

Missing from the life I crave. The life I worked so hard for. The life I deserve to live.

We are not hysterical. We are not exaggerating. Exercise has not healed us. And this is not all in our heads.

Long COVID exists, and so do we.

Many like me have spent countless days gone; I speak for us all when I say we refuse to be forgotten.

Three Months Going on Four

Andrew David King

So pain's a lousier archer
now. His trick is curved
by pills I feed
not to myself but to the black
statue of pain in me. It works,
it doesn't, the reed
around the tooth, the waves
of ache smoothing my hull.
Two crows on the antenna
know what transmits what:
the roof's palette
of lichen runs in place, ledgers
of snow resolve
their balance into air. My breath
here changes nothing there.
Boots, somewhere in the building,
hunt their echoes
in ten paces. If you flinch you cause
the moon to swerve,
as all else you do, though nonc
can see or tell: as I stand
in the deluge with my spoon.

Icarus in Convalescence

Andrew David King

Above the slick stars of the aloe vera
whose arms propped up a leaden tent of heat,
she moved as would a rattler past the chairs
where strangers plumed their strangenesses at tea

to find him there: his torso ornamental,
his calves turned driftwood, stone shorn by the sea.
How far had he from the sun's retina fallen,
scanned by the shallow eyes of buckeye seeds—

infrared puddle, coldness-of-the-summer:
she robed him in robe after robe of names.
Adrift past death, he found his life redundant,
vultures and sparrows chanting in his brain.

But turned onto his back, from within scar-gloss,
new bone thrust through the mud and graveyard moss.

All Good on Paper

Andrew David King

I'm all good on paper:
the test is clean. Neighbor's got
a white square fired
in blue December. I'm all
goodness and truth, nothing
the MRI's eye could glean.
And yet, in my chest, a fire
three Tylenol crackle in:
sparks writing with bright
longhand what's read
once and gone. I'm all good
on paper, he says, so don't
see me again. There's no need.

You have the catalpa trees,
an attic rank with books,
and tea. You're all good on paper.
Look at what writes on me:
our headlights chase down
asphalt in the valley, yank
blankness's blanket from any
random animal. The ground
recedes
into the perfection of not
being seen. So like this pain
and me. Silent *tick tick tick*
in the dark tumbleweed.

Still Life with Dead Passion Fruit Vine and Dog Bowl

Andrew David King

Introducing ourselves to the moral philosopher
on Zoom, my father vacuuming in the background,
my heart jumped the high-dive once
and once and once and once and once again.
I mean by this nothing metaphorical.
If I died then I didn't know it: I woke from a dream
of birth into another where the Capitol is still,
as the weatherpeople say, stormed, where a karst mountain,
like a shoulder blade tenting skin, still snares
a fisher-poet's mind. With its skirt of mist
it seems not to be another of the earth's tired organs
after all. So there is no need to flee
to the parade of off-duty cashiers with their skates
and boomboxes to feel as though life might delude
itself again. No need for the Babels of tangerines
in grocery stores to fret and callus. The fluorescents
will hold the memory of their shock for a human
second and then quiet down into the solitude of milk.
Our joy, and not the sand in the chute, rubs us red.
The mockingbirds, expecting us, don't flinch.

Limbo

Michele Black

ESSAY

I started a new part-time job on the third anniversary of my COVID-19 infection. For 15 hours a week, I cared for animals at a small refuge in New Mexico, feeding, training, cleaning, and cuddling them — all totally manageable activities. However, the 300-yard walk up a rocky hill to the animal facilities at least three times a day was not included in the job description. Within a week, I was back to sleeping most of the nonwork hours, experiencing tremors and anxiety. After six weeks, I was a wreck and regretfully gave my notice. My expectations exceeded my physical abilities. I think it's safe to say that my working days are over, which is a shame because my savings are running dry. I am back to square one, not well enough to work, yet not sick enough to qualify for assistance. I am in limbo.

I used to make a living as an artist, creating in my mobile studio, traveling to art shows, and selling to galleries and online. In March 2020, that all changed. While camped deep in the Sonoran desert, I became too sick to contemplate driving to a medical facility. For about a week, I thought I might simply die there in my sleep, as it required a conscious effort to breathe. Gradually, the breathing difficulty passed, but I was left with a terrible cough and a sense of wonder at my survival. I felt OK but diminished.

Had the illness even been the virus? Nobody knew anything at that point.

I dusted myself off and began driving to a show in California with a new collection of small sculptures. While I was en route, the governor closed all public events, and that was that.

Over the next couple of months, I traveled back to Idaho and began to experience some very peculiar symptoms. I had strange internal vibrations, like something moving inside my body. I couldn't catch my breath and had crushing fatigue. Multiple times a day, I needed to lie down and pass out. Other symptoms included heart pounding and palpitations, sleep apnea, sudden sensitivities to food, hair loss, and brain fog. Brain fog deserves a far more sinister name. It sounds misty and quiet, but in reality it is a dense stupor of confusion. The traits that I thought of as "me" evaporated. I felt like one of those zombie beetles limping along after death. Just who was driving this bus anyway?

Nobody wanted to hear the tedious details of my mysterious ailment. My grown kids, who live far away, listened with sympathy, but, let's face it, chronic anything is a bore, so I didn't give it top conversational billing. One friend thought long-haul COVID was something that afflicted truckers. Another questioned whether I had truly had COVID-19 or was inventing it. I was offered a lot of advice: push through, toughen up, go for a run. Quite a few friends drifted away in the process, particularly the ones who stood by such comments as "We refuse to live in fear" or "It's just the flu."

I also parted ways with those who were quietly anti-vaccine but didn't tell anyone. I can thank one of those friends for my second infection! I guess I should have asked about their vaccination status before we had dessert together.

Thankfully, my second bout with COVID was not as terrible as the first, likely because I had a six-month-old Johnson & Johnson vaccine going for me. Stories circulated that Long COVID improved with the vaccines, but I saw no change. I got the booster, then the bivalent booster, and I will keep getting them. They may have played a role in my recovery, but possibly not. I'm not taking any chances.

I have survived camping alone for the better part of three years now. I have sold my tools, display supplies, show tent, and the occasional piece of art to keep myself afloat.

But real support came from a few nonpublic Facebook groups dedicated to Long COVID. Members of those groups compared notes on symptoms, meds, and supplements and held each other's hands. I learned from them about low histamine diets, pacing, and post-exertional malaise (PEM). This is another misnamed condition: PEM demands that I rest between activities, or else, the Crash. The pattern looks like this: do the dishes, lay down; shower, nap; get groceries, sleep for a day.

Long-term improvements can be hard to notice when you're busy dealing with the small stuff of living with chronic illness, but I enrolled in an ongoing study with Johns Hopkins, which has helped me track my recovery. Thirty months post-infection, I woke up one morning feeling like my old self. Naturally, feeling energized, I tried to do everything. Big mistake. But it was still a beacon of hope. Over time, more good days came, and though I would pay for it the next day, eventually I was able to walk a mile again.

I am back to making art, house- and pet-sitting, and appreciating the great outdoors. I am not sure I will ever fully recover, but I will get by. And that still feels like living in limbo.

Three Years and Counting

Jessica B. Sokol

ESSAY

Illness strikes me in February 2020, after returning home from a holiday in Ireland. When I catch up in person with a pal who had been vacationing in Colorado, he shares that his girlfriend became can't-get-out-of-bed ill on their trip. The following day, I wake up with a high fever, chills, a sore throat, and labored breathing. I can't swallow food, keep water down, or shower without fainting. I have this unshakable migraine and a cough that stabs at my ribs and my back. Friends in Ireland phone to report identical symptoms. My husband, Joel, a flight attendant, flies home, and my parents, who live nearby, care for me. This lasts two weeks and is never diagnosed.

A month later, COVID becomes an ominous cloud on the horizon, rabidly swirling in the air. I can't know if I had already gotten it by then, and we still aren't sure, but there was little doubt in my mind; I hadn't been sick since food poisoning on a Barcelona business trip in 2016.

In March, I'm living in a downtown apartment complex and working in international education. Joel's and my careers indefinitely halt and we're suddenly living together full-time, something we've never done because we're usually on the road. With COVID everywhere now, our typically cozy and welcoming apartment feels suffocating. The tenants are making everything worse: they loiter 24/7, block entrances and fire escapes, prevent us from safely going outside. They throw parties, break locks to private entrances, and rip fire extinguishers off walls. Others are smoking, which is strictly prohibited. My calls to the property manager fall on deaf ears. The disturbing sound of nonstop hacking in the middle of the night is a visceral noise seeping through windows and walls. It's especially haunting since I'd been so sick so recently. Joel and I vigilantly stay indoors, not wanting to risk anything. I have trouble breathing on several occasions and feel a near-constant exhaustion. I chalk it up to stress.

In August, I wake up violently ill again with a 104-degree fever. The entire right side of my upper body is in unbearable pain. My primary care physician won't see me because of COVID. He instructs me to go to our hospital respiratory center for tests and X-rays. Joel has to carry me down our apartment stairs. It turns out I have pleurisy, a lung infection, and pneumonia. My COVID test is negative, but my doctor still won't see me because he says there are too many false negatives going around.

A prescription inhaler, antibiotics, and Lorazepam don't make me feel any better. I revisit the respiratory center, where another round of antibiotics causes intense stomach pain. There are nights I can't catch my breath when Joel cradles me on the bathroom floor. It takes two months to recover. Family and friends, including infectious disease doctors and hospital nurses, suspect I suffer from Long COVID. I think everything will heal; I'll be OK. But I'm not.

In June, I'm fully vaxxed and feeling better, but not going out in public and ever cautious in our apartment building. Joel and I are at my parents' celebrating Father's Day when I start coughing up blood. He rushes me to the ER, which is inundated with COVID. The vaccine has been available for a few months, but there aren't enough rooms or doctors in a hospital with sick unvaccinated patients everywhere.

I'm hooked up to all sorts of tubes in the ER, waiting for more X-rays and more tests. I need a bronchoscopy. Something is very wrong with my right lung, but the staff are bombarded and can't tell me when it could happen. The hemoptysis becomes worse. Days and nights pass, and still no one is available to perform my overdue procedure. So, my body takes a dangerous turn. I start throwing up and choking on blood everywhere I go, from the CT room floor to the operating table. I can't lie down or breathe. That's the last thing I remember for a while.

Nothing makes sense when I wake up in the ICU several days later. Initially, I can't move any part of my body. When I'm strong enough to hold my phone, I have hundreds of unread texts and dozens of missed calls. The most disconcerting thing I see, though, is the date. My dad is next to me, and I ask him what day it is.

He responds, "Sweetie, you know you were in a medically induced coma? You were intubated on a ventilator." I didn't know.

"See, you're the 'interesting case' in the hospital, and you never want to be the 'interesting case' in a hospital," one pulmonologist says. He can't tell me if this is related to my post Ireland sickness. Though between that and a newly diagnosed autoimmune condition, he thinks, I could have been brewing the perfect storm to cause what I have now, which is a severely-infected lung cavity that wasn't treated in time. I feel like my life isn't real to me. How could it be when I just learned that I'd been on life support at 37?

Joel and my parents spend as many hours as they're allowed with me in the ICU. We begin a long healing journey together after my 12 days in the hospital. They help me lift a fork, take me to the bathroom, and patiently stand by my side as I learn to walk again. I start remembering the days and nights alone in the hospital; the hallucinations of spiders under the bed, the locusts at the window, and a graphically sweaty threesome happening next to me. And I recall the real nightmares of shitting in bedpans, having the tube pulled from my throat, a blood transfusion, the IVs in every inch of my neck and arms. I remember waking up with my long blond hair in braids and feeling like straw, not knowing who washed it. The extreme loneliness, and the terror, keeps washing over me.

In July and after I leave the hospital, Joel and I stay at my parent's house until we can move out of our apartment and into a small home in a nearby farming community. We can't live downtown anymore; too risky. We hire movers for the heavy lifting and Joel cleans the space. I don't get to bid farewell to a home that I took care of for eight years because there are too many safety hazards, physical and psychological. Plus, I can't even walk up the stairs.

I suffer waves of post-traumatic stress and crippling anxiety. The lung cavity still hasn't shrunk and I have difficulty breathing. My months are filled with doctor appointments, CT scans, blood tests, physical therapy, fear-ridden flashbacks, panic attacks, and nightmares.

Having an "up" day during these stressful isolated times is rare, but with this respiratory condition, I can't afford to contract any kind of virus. I must vet everyone I spend time with, and unlike most people, I can't just move on from COVID, even being fully boosted. I still haven't been around loved ones with sniffling kids or entered a grocery store.

After another February goes by, I've missed out on a full year of adventures, family Thanksgiving, book readings, and holiday parties. It's difficult to digest. I'm advised these are not low-risk events for me, but this isn't getting easier. The fear of getting sick again is all-encompassing, so watching the world pass me by is my new shitty normal. While this doesn't bode well for my natural extroverted tendencies and love for travel, I adapt to this reclusive lifestyle. I spend many days bingeing Anthony Bourdain reruns just to feel alive. My job now is trying to stay healthy, to heal.

Joel becomes my caregiver, the sole bill-payer, and our therapist, all in addition to being my husband. He retires from the airlines and now works full-time from home for a health insurance company. Hanging above his office chair is a magnetic world map full of colorful pins and unforgettable memories from all of the countries we traveled to together. It looks like a stopped clock, with no new pins added since our Ireland trip. Our lifetime flight benefits will have to wait.

I think it's a minor miracle that Joel is still deeply attracted to me. He proves time and again that he outwardly craves me and wants to make love after all he's seen. Even so, my vulnerable body sometimes doesn't feel like mine because it's been through so much.

It's frustrating to see the invincibility many feel now, and I hope that these thoughts about people's insensitivity will not turn into more stories I'll feel compelled to write one day. It's getting harder to accept these last years filled with COVID and such an unknown future. I hold back tears with a lipstick-stained smile, trying to hide the pain of this long haul.

Sometimes Not Always

Mary Ladd

ESSAY

When a new primary care provider proclaims that Long COVID is *real*, when I finally feel seen and heard, I fantasize about clapping and exclaiming, "Yay! Yay! Yay!" I might've acted on such a spontaneous reaction in the before times. Instead — now — I hunch over. Familiar, fearful questions simmer.

What is going on with my exhausted body? Will I ever feel better? How will I pay my bills?

"I just saw a much younger patient. Her systems are destroyed. Like you," says this lady doctor.

Um, thanks?!

Walking home, I see people presumably on their way to work, walking much faster than I can. Another question comes up:

Is there something I can do to feel better when I wake up each day?

Long COVID feels the worst in the morning. Sometimes — not always — it's as if a baker's dozen of incredibly strong and fit baby gnomes have hammered my neck, legs, and skull nonsexually throughout the night.

Sometimes — not always — in the following hours, other Long COVID symptoms and adjacent potential conditions wreak havoc: pinching pain and nerve damage; missing vocab words; food sensitivities via mast cell activation syndrome; insomnia; fatigue; bubbling, twitching, rushing sensations in body parts that should not bubble, twitch, and rush; swollen and cloudy eyes; a broken vagina, broken butthole, broken guts; spinning and nausea and dizziness. Half my vagina went fully numb at one point. Another time, I swear microscopic bugs were crawling in and around all of my private parts.

Am I in a science fiction film?

When pulling on underwear or pants hurts, I wince and sob, getting ready to see the OB-GYN. There, the team listens and probes. Yet, ultimately, I don't get what I want: a "COVID vagina" chart designation to prove how wackadoodle my vagina has become. Instead, the medical verdict is that the tissues down there are thin. Maybe it's a win-win not to have crabs.

Sexual dysfunction and other bummer symptoms are familiar after a triple-negative breast cancer diagnosis 10 years ago. I remember fantasizing about sleeping because I felt depressed at how cancer obliterated my energy and enthusiasm. I'd sometimes — not always — pine for pre-cancer routines revolving around eating, family, event work, and food writing.

Scavenging for leftovers at work revved me up. My mouth would water, and there would be a tingling desire from anticipating the exact moment when it was possible to hunt and gather tasty treats expertly: a pallet of charcuterie, squeeze bottles of delectable gourmet sauces, a flat of mixed greens, or a three-pound wheel of gooey cheese. Depending on how an event's guests ate, I'd spot and track items of interest back to the kitchen. Packing away any pleasing personal haul, however, often turned into more of a group experience: The crew would divvy up rations and head into the night sweaty and happy with overstuffed bags of shrink-wrapped savory tarts, tan to-go boxes, and a pointy Acme baguette or three. A fierce adrenaline rush resumed the following day when I pawed through the fridge, debating what to pair with what.

I was an adventurous eater long before I ate calf brains on camera with Anthony Bourdain. Breast cancer upended my exciting eating days. Medical pros and well-meaning friends told me about the connection between inflammation and diet, with the annoying suggestion that I should cut back on booze, sugar, meat, or the rest of the rich foods. In my Long COVID era, cautious eating seems wise because of new-to-me histamine-related allergic reactions. I can't ditch my lifetime habits because food still represents joy, togetherness, and fun. Foods now irritate my entire being with headaches, scratchy throats, and worse. I'm facing an ongoing question of if-when-how I can ghost a growing list: cocoa, vinegar, caffeine, pizza, chocolate, wheat bread, mushrooms, dairy, spinach, and the perennial favorite, Sriracha. Even citrus sometimes — not always — puffs up my throat and eyes. I can't fake being vibrant, normal, and attractive with four rounds of hiccups, bloating, heart palpitations, and loud funneling and whirring noises — as if a small bird has taken over — in my right ear. It should be against the law to have diarrhea and constipation in the same afternoon!

I can't keep it all straight, given worse pressing symptoms. What is anti-inflammatory? What is low-histamine? It's confusing that some fruits and veggies now cause harmful reactions. Figuring out Long COVID treatment, pills, and ingredients is pure Whack-a-Mole. Researching, prepping, and storing food could be a full-time job. I'm supposed to rest when I feel terrible, but I often can't.

Hope floats the same as turds.

Long COVID sneakily enrobes me in molasses, nullifying timelines and plans. It slows everything down, from breathing to the ability to think, move, or even walk. I start daydreaming about stretching out on my oversized blue couch. Sometimes — not always — when the back of my eyes feel roasted from the inside, or a nasty claw grips the lower spine, I try to remember it's just what's on the Long COVID menu for today.

Early scans showed no lung damage, though I sometimes — not always — feel breathlessness on the edge of choking. When I want a good laugh, I flash back to one online recommendation to freeze cooked food immediately or throw out leftovers because the harmful histamine levels grow the longer cooked food sits. But I love leftovers! One treasured favorite remains a still-warm, fragrant rotisserie chicken accompanied by dips, salads, slaws, noodles, and freshly chopped herbs. In the before times, I got in touch with my inner glutton by gobbling piece after piece in the grocery store parking lot. Now, rotisserie chicken shouldn't cross my lips because its life under that deli heat lamp may lead to higher histamines, and thus, a decent chance that I'll have a headache and uncomfortable throat tickle just a few bites in.

Who has time for this?

Bountiful food symbolizes TLC. I feel like a rebel endlessly scrolling pictures of extra-large purple ube cookies, decadent Detroit-style pizza squares, or a laminated buttery pastry with endless chocolate and hazelnut layers. Let's give the Red Bay Coffee employee responsible for that masterpiece a raise and round of jazz hands!

Sometimes — not always — just walking from my front door to the car is tough. I can't imagine attending events or going to the office as I used to. Even a new travel drugstore eye mask represents another modern dilemma and mindfuck. Who do I talk to about this flammable contraption with microbeads that kill dolphins and likely cause cancer? I'll stick with my bag of frozen green beans that gets used so often to calm my skin that the label has rubbed off. These Long COVID skin issues seem more appropriate for a lizard than a middle-aged lady. When the tiny blisters colonize my arm, I feel guilty and ashamed of how they ooze. In colder months, different mountain ranges of bumps erupt and disappear from my neck and legs. One morning, my foot twitches and itches: The entire layer of skin on the top and sides of my foot gently and quickly sloughs off into a disgusting translucent pile on the floor.

Should dead skin be composted or put in the garbage? Asking for a friend!

Sometimes — not always — insecurity is just under the surface. Losing a full head of hair to cancer woke me to how much I identified with shiny auburn locks. When the punishing Red Devil chemo iced through my nearly collapsed veins, it seemed superficial to ache for the normalcy that longer hair represented. Two months into COVID-19, female pattern baldness returned. Spying strands lying between two eggs in a carton brings home the irony of loss against the literal symbol of fertility and nutrition. I still have significant scalp gaps, but I'm grateful that my height lets me hide the follicle situation artfully.

How many strands are left?

Sometimes — not always — a coughing routine takes over at night before a jewel-colored dispensary gummy kicks in. I cover my top half with a heavy laptop pillow for a budget-weight-blanket vibe. Visualizing being wrapped in a blanket suited just to me is something I've steadily done since I had cancer. I used to swaddle my son in a blanket like an adorable baby burrito, my stomach quietly rumbling. When Long COVID insomnia tortures me, I imagine the grandmas I met on writing assignments wrapping me in soft corn husks. Turning into a tamale calms me better than any app, and my eyes quickly become heavy. Instead of worrying about life and symptoms, I feel cozy and secure, like everything could be OK. There is still a bigger world beyond this, even if I am anxious and unsure of what's possible. On other nights, my brain serves up sepia-colored films of childhood gatherings around pizza, an equally strong representation of love. I am rich in experiences that comfort me. Even bad pizza is pizza, like bad sex is sex — you still have it.

Am I dreaming of my birthday party or wake?

Neuropathy shivers like angry soda bubbles traveling to my toes and feet. Nightly vibrations whoosh through my ears and head. Waking up with heavy dead hands, I pretend to dive into a giant salad spinner to work this painful static out. Navigating extensive unknowns is scary. "Please hire a hit man to surprise-shoot me if I become too sick from this," cues a sad, awkward moment with my spouse.

With a once again broken body, I am limited on if, how, and when I can engage with the world. One massive difference between the uncertainty of early-stage aggressive breast cancer is that then, I had more hope of a firm endpoint, even if chemo and so many surgeries had painful and scary lasting effects. Long COVID remains a constant without clear answers and options for me and millions. Sometimes — not always — I just focus on the activities and tools that can bring ease and comfort to others. Since food equals love, maybe we can book a global potluck party.

I'll order the pizza!

A Mate for Life

Alexis Misko

ESSAY

In the winter of 2021, newly disabled by a COVID infection at age 33, I learned that bald eagles mate for life.

For six months, I could do little more than lie still in a silent, neurological haze, curtains drawn, my husband offering to paint my toenails to interact with me. He prepared my meals, managed the household, washed my hair, and dumped out my urine, trying to fill the enormous new gaps in our life with small joys whenever possible. We mourned deeply for all that might never be.

When I was finally able to sustain looking at a television or computer screen, I went searching for easy, soothing content, like animals in nature, reveling in their vibrant aliveness during my profound isolation, wishing I could instead hear their rustles and calls in person, dirt on my boots and sweating among vernal greenery. I discovered a 24-hour livestream of a bald eagle's nest in northeast Florida; checking it became a daily ritual.

Once paired, bald eagles return each season to the same nest, unless their mate dies, for their average life span of 20 to 30 years. I watched as a parent eagle tenderly fed two wrinkly gray heaps of fuzz bloody fish guts from its beak, their reptilian eyelids groggy. Staggering around my kitchen feeling poisoned, I clung to the counter while standing for the two agonizing minutes it took to heat water for tea, limbs numb and heart racing. I learned that eagles have a locking mechanism in their talons that allows them to stay securely upright while sleeping, an astounding feat for someone with exhaustion, muscle weakness, and insomnia. The eaglets bobbled and toppled, eventually expanding in size and gaining balance, leaping out of the nest in a phenomenon known as branching.

I went outside to sit on my porch for the first time, yet I could only stay there briefly. I sobbed at the smell of the neighbor's freshly cut grass and the breeze on my face. When it rained, white peeked out from underneath the black feathers on the fledglings' heads, though they would not fully resemble adult bald eagles for five years. One became stuck on a branch below the nest, endlessly squawking at its sibling as if pleading for aid, wings repeatedly flapping upward in determination, though only enough to graze the camera lens. I rode in a car for the first time in 15 months, nauseated and stiff with pain, once familiar landmarks surrealistic after living in seclusion.

I watched the eagles from the first egg pipping and hatching in January to spring, when the juveniles were strong enough to perch upright and gaze out at the horizon, preening, anticipating. In May, the first young eagle flew away.

"When will I get my wings back?" I asked my husband.

He squeezed my hand. "I don't know," he said. "But I'll be here."

Outside, sounds of nighttime hung, near but desperately inaccessible: train whistles, car tires, people on the sidewalk talking and laughing freedom. I watched a lightning bug crawl across the windowsill from the couch, glowing, waiting to fly. —

Reading Group Guide

These questions aim to foster deeper understanding and empathy while stimulating discussion, reflection, and possible action.

Which story or piece resonated with you the most and why?

Can you identify the emotions that were common across the different narratives? How did these emotions impact you as a reader?

Do you or someone close to you have experience with Long COVID? How does that compare to what you read in the book?

How has your perception of Long COVID deepened or changed after reading these personal experiences from those dealing with it?

What role does resting, sleep, and fatigue play in these narratives?

In which ways do the poems provide a different perspective on the patient experience compared with the stories?

How do you view spaces such as home, work, and medical facilities differently?

Can you draw any parallels between the struggles described in the book and other hardships you've encountered in life?

Which of the authors or characters did you empathize with the most and why?

How do you think societal stigma affects people with Long COVID, based on the narratives?

In what ways does the creative approach of the authors contribute to our understanding of Long COVID?

What insights have you gained about resilience and hope?

Have you ever used writing and journaling to navigate your own serious illness or another tough situation? If so, what was that like?

How has reading this book affected your understanding of the broader impact of the COVID-19 pandemic?

What actions or changes interest you after reading these stories and poems?

How can we better support individuals with Long COVID, based on what you've learned from this book?

Remember, each voice in this book represents someone's lived reality. May their experiences inspire action to support and advocate for the growing worldwide Long COVID community.

Writing Prompts

These writing prompts are our gift to you. Try them out on your own or build community by sharing and listening to what others create in a small group setting.

Guidelines: Studies show that writing things down is deeply therapeutic. If you are newer to writing, at first, it may be tough and possibly surprising when certain thoughts and emotions surface. Write what you can. Keep the pen or pencil to the paper, or fingers on the keyboard, for five or 10 minutes as a start. If you stumble, write a list of words, thoughts and ideas that you can come back to. There's no need to fuss over spelling or word flow. This writing is for you, but you may decide to later share it with the world in some fashion.

Writing Tips: Try writing as if you are in conversation with a close friend, favorite teacher, or other trusted person.

Characters: Perhaps you want to do a deep dive into the details for your narrator or character(s), which can turn into a description of what they are wearing and the shape of their features. There's also the chance to dive in and note what possibly makes them tick including likes, dislikes, joys, and sorrows.

Who is near your narrator or character(s), and what are they doing? What is the history of the place and people, and how have things changed from a century ago, decade ago, year ago, and even month ago? Detail how people move and talk, including height, posture, voice, and mannerisms. What colors, textures, people and things are nearby? Shading, colors, and scents are especially evocative.

Era: Does the action take place today? Last year? Your childhood? The future? Or a different time or world?

Genre: Write a story, poem, fiction, or whatever strikes your fancy!

Use the following prompts to guide your writing:

Prompt One: Imagine a conversation with COVID-19. What would you like to say to it? Write for 10-12 minutes.

Then, if in a small group setting, participants who feel comfortable can share their writing and discuss their feelings and experiences.

Prompt Two: Describe a day in your life before 2020. Compare it with a day in your life now. What has changed? What has remained the same? Write for 12-15 minutes.

Prompt Three: Describe your perfect day. What are you doing? Who are you with?

Prompt Four: Write about a time when you felt particularly loved, strong and/or capable.

Prompt Five: Write a letter to your immune system. What would you like to say to it?

If in a small group setting, participants who feel comfortable can share their writing and discuss their thoughts, feelings, and experiences.

Reflect for a few minutes: What have you learned today about yourself and your life? Draw, doodle, think quietly, breathe. While closing your writing session, remember to be gentle with yourself, since new memories and thoughts may come up over the next few days.

Congratulations. Keep writing, we are rooting for you!

A Conversation with Founding Editor Mary Ladd

Tell us about your background as a writer and connection to Long COVID.

I've done a lot of food writing, essays, and copywriting. My writing changed when I had breast cancer 10 years ago and began to focus more on health issues with a book project called *The Wig Diaries*, illustrated by *San Francisco Chronicl*e cartoonist Don Asmussen. Using dark humor, that book helped explain the truth about the nitty-gritty details of what life is like when you're immunocompromised, and sometimes invisible to society. Humor remains a coping mechanism and tool I use for creative work and daily life.

Having the most severe form of breast cancer at a young age helped me understand what it's like to be afraid in the middle of the night, vulnerable, and need help from society and others. So when I contracted COVID in 2022, followed by lingering Long COVID symptoms, it was quite similar to breast cancer in that it brought up a lot of the same fears and vulnerabilities. How will I pay my bills? How can I continue to show up as a human, writer, parent, and spouse? With brain fog and fatigue, I can't be as physically active, and must say no to so many things. I'm often stuck in bed and working from home. I never know when Long COVID is going to overwhelm my body and yank me out of whatever it is I'm doing or planning.

I've done a lot of healing through writing and taught people how to process their trauma or illness in that way. I know how healing it can be for me, whether or not something gets published. I like using writing to help others feel less alone, but also to teach them about something they might not have experienced themselves. I'm not alone with COVID since there's a wider community out there.

Can you talk about your vision for Long Hauler Publishing and your original inspiration for the project?

The Long COVID Reader is the first of many books. The vision is to allow writers, whether they have professional experience or not, to share as many stories as possible so they can reach people all over the world. Long Hauler Publishing is meant to be part of the large community that is made by and for long haulers. We are also adjacent to people who have conditions such as ME/CFS and other immunocompromised and disabling conditions. They are our family members, our sisters and brothers, so to speak. I have usually said yes to opportunities and collaborators and plan on bringing people together, online or through hybrid events. Future books will feature international contributors, and we can pair that with more group writing sessions and handouts.

I hope Long Hauler Publishing mirrors my experience contributing to a breast cancer publication for the young breast cancer community called *Wildfire Magazine*, which is founded and run by April Stearns. She helps so many people with breast cancer. I wanted to do the same for the Long COVID community. At *Wildfire* reading events, I feel seen and heard. Whenever I receive a *Wildfire* newsletter on my phone, I read the whole thing immediately. Start to finish, which is rare. I attend the events and read the magazine as soon as humanly possible because it helps me feel less afraid and alone. So that's what Long Hauler Publishing hopes to achieve. I'd like to encourage as many people as possible to learn, write, create, read, and support each other.

Why do you think this project is especially important right now?

COVID-19 was arguably the most serious societal disruption in over a century. This project is important right now because masking has largely disappeared. We need to remind gatekeepers, politicians, researchers, and those in power that, no matter what they think or believe, Long COVID has not gone away. There's a huge number of people stuck, suffering, and unable to work or properly participate in their own lives. They need disability payments, housing assistance, support for food, nutrition, caregiving, and parenting.

Humanizing illness and people who are immunocompromised is critical because if it doesn't affect you or your immediate circle, you likely don't consider it. The Long COVID Reader is the first of its kind, the first to offer creative and literary insight into the long hauler slice of life. A lot of these stories make me cry, nod with recognition, and even laugh. Frankly, these folks aren't meant to inspire anyone. We're not heroes. I'm a jerk, believe me, but you should know I'm here and my condition exists.

What sort of readers will appreciate this anthology?

Anyone who is curious about Long COVID or wonders whether or not they have Long COVID will get something out of this anthology. There are 200 symptoms and counting, and it's a mixed bag. Additionally, parents, family members, friends, and caregivers of those with Long COVID will find value in these pages. Long haulers can't exactly present a document to those who care about them and say, "Read my mind. This is what I need," but this anthology will shed some light on their experiences.

Those in the medical research community seem eager to read this one because it offers those in the medical field insight into their patients and research subjects. Medical practitioners may be working hard while playing catch up.

Finally, this anthology will also appeal to people who simply love wonderful literary offerings, as well as poetry.

What are some logistical risks and challenges from publishing this book?
We work with folks who are immunocompromised, so there may be some delays in communication. Using the word "COVID" might also create a barrier for us, given the level of misinformation about COVID-19 online and in the broader world. This book does not provide medical advice. It's simply a slice of life and creative expression provided by long haulers.

What do you envision for the future of Long Hauler Publishing?
Maybe Long Hauler Publishing can expand to become a nonprofit as inspired by an important website called *Who We Lost: A Portable COVID Memorial*, run by Martha Greenwald. She is a writing instructor who has provided a space, book, and tool kit for people who want to tell stories about those who died from COVID-19 during the pandemic. I would love to provide similar tool kits so people with Long COVID can be creative, regardless of their location and socioeconomic status. There will also be more writing sessions, classes, and events. I'd like to grow so we're not a shoestring operation and partner with as many Long COVID organizations as possible while continuing to expand the team.

This project brings me so much joy. I wake up a lot earlier than I used to, but that could also be yet another Long COVID bodily response. There's a sense of purpose because it helps a growing group of people. With all my catering and event planning experience plus writing, I've been preparing for this project and effort my whole life. I'm so moved by those who submitted their work and overly grateful that we've been able to scale quickly. When people say "Yes!" instead of "How are you going to do that?," it's great.

About the Contributors

Adrienne Asher was born in San Francisco, California, where her college studies focused on creative writing and fine arts. Many of her poems explore ways of finding what female agency and power look like personally, in mythology, and in history. She is published in numerous anthologies and journals, including *Bellingham Review, The Laurel Review,* and Black Mountain Press' *The 64 Best Poets of 2018*. She lives in the Pacific Northwest with her musician partner, a Maine Coon cat, and nine miles of books.

Rachel R. Baum contracted COVID-19 in March 2020. She is the editor of *Funeral & Memorial Service Readings Poems & Tributes* (McFarland, 1999) and author of the blog *Bark: Confessions of a Dog Trainer*. As a long hauler, she founded the Saratoga Peace Pod, began writing poetry, and created the position of Poet Laureate for Saratoga Springs, New York.

Ellen Belluomini MacKenzie, PhD, is an associate professor at the University of Massachusetts Global. She contracted COVID-19 twice, leading to her struggles with Long COVID. She is a mixed-media artist and social worker.

Michele Black is a roving metalsmith/sculptor hailing from Ketchum, Idaho. A full-time RVer since 2015, art, reading, microgardens, and food preservation are her favorite pursuits.

Brian Burke was born and raised in Illinois, where he still resides. Brian is disabled with autism, PTSD, heatstroke sensitivity, Long COVID damage, and other problems, but currently runs the YouTube show *ARTSAGANZA*, where he works with others to promote various multimedia and unknown artists.

Lisa Carpentier is a United States Postal Service employee.

David Charles Braun was a volunteer fireman for 12 years. He then worked as a safety inspector/ contractor, but he had to quit his job of 22 years due to COVID-19. He is an avid outdoorsman who enjoys fishing, camping, and birdwatching.

Austin Crowley is a writer from Connecticut, formerly based in Brooklyn, New York. His work has been featured in *The Inkwell* and *From Arthur's Seat.* He is currently in the Master's in Creative Writing program at University of Edinburgh. His Long COVID began in March 2020, and he has since developed POTS.

Pato Hebert is an artist, teacher, and organizer. He is also a COVID-19 long hauler, living with the ongoing impacts of the coronavirus since March 2020 and publicly addressing the pandemic through creativity and community building. Hebert serves as Chair and teaches in the Department of Art & Public Policy at New York University Tisch School of the Arts.

Emily Fraser is a documentary filmmaker, teacher, and writer based in Oakland, California. She has ME/CFS, MCAS, and POTS, and has been housebound since a COVID-like virus in March 2020. Emily holds a bachelor's degree in environmental policy and art from the College of William and Mary and an MFA in documentary film and video from Stanford University.

Candis Freeman Johnson is a 40-year-old African American woman who contracted COVID-19 during the first wave in August 2020. Due to chronic pain, she works flexible gigs like substitute teaching, Uber, and remote jobs that do not require a strict schedule. She loves to travel, bake desserts, thrift-shop, spend quality time with her daughters at the park feeding ducks, research fashion, be creative, and be active.

Cynthia Gardner's poetry has been published in several journals and anthologies. Her chapbook, *How Will They Find Me*, was a finalist in the 2012 Finishing Line Press chapbook competition. She is in her 48th year as a clinical social worker in The Berkshires of Massachusetts. She has not tasted food since December 2019, when she was very sick for over two weeks.

Sonya Huber is the author of eight books, including the new guide, *Voice First: A Writer's Manifesto* and the award-winning essay collection on chronic pain, *Pain Woman Takes Your Keys*. Her essay collection, *Love and Industry: A Midwestern Workbook*, was published in September 2023. She teaches at Fairfield University and in the Fairfield low-residency MFA program.

Anastasia Jill (she/they) is a queer writer living in Central Florida. She has been battling Long COVID since late 2022 and advocates for elevating voices of the chronically ill in the arts. Her work has been featured or is upcoming with *Poets.org, Sundog Lit, Pithead Chapel, Contemporary Verse 2, OxMag, Broken Pencil*, and more.

Abigail Koppes, PhD, is an associate professor of engineering in Boston, where her group studies nervous system and gut disorders. She caught mild COVID-19 in March of 2020 and Long Covid neuralgia in the summer of 2021. Prior to LC she enjoyed travel, extreme sports, hiking, running, and spending time with her husband and two huskies.

Jennifer Kreatsoulas, PhD, is an author and certified yoga therapist specializing in eating disorders. She is the author of *The Courageous Path to Healing* (Llewellyn Worldwide, 2022), and her writing has been featured widely in print, broadcast, and online media. She has been living with Long COVID since November 2020.

Maya Lea is a former museum curator, educator, and placemaker. She has edited and ghostwritten numerous works of both fiction and nonfiction, including a groundbreaking art history text. She first contracted COVID-19 in April 2020.

Steven Lewis was the first person in Port Royal, South Carolina, to be hospitalized with the scourge. He spent a harrowing week in the ICU followed by almost three years of cycling symptoms. A torrent of writings have come out of this experience.

Rowan MacDonald was diagnosed with Long COVID in 2022 and became a writer soon after. He loves the escapism that writing provides. When not writing, he enjoys spending time with his dog, sipping cups of tea, and reading the words of others.

Kristy Malone is a Long COVID survivor, Licensed Marriage and Family Therapist, and business owner. Kristy runs a free monthly support group, serves as a therapist for long haulers, and maintains a COVID-safe office. Kristy wants other long haulers to know that everyone heals on their own timeline, and to never give up on yourself.

Sabrina McQueen Johnson, PhD, is a wife, mother, and retired school principal with over 26 years of experience as an educator. Dr. Johnson's educational studies include journalism and educational leadership, policy, and law. However, it is her personal relationship with God she values most. She is a Christian woman who believes in the power of prayer and enjoys writing, reading, traveling, and sharing the word of God.

Mary Jo Mettler, LPC, was born and raised on the Kenai Peninsula in Alaska. She was diagnosed with COVID-19 on November 12, 2020. She loves Jesus, the people he's blessed her life with, animals, mountain views, the colors orange and purple, miniatures, and making others laugh.

Patricia Milano is a COVID-19 survivor and long hauler of three years. She has been in the veterans' homeless shelter in Boston for over seven months and her dog is in foster care with an agency that is going to reunite them soon. Due to COVID-19, she has lost all of her personal belongings, a place to live, and almost her life. She is still struggling but is very grateful to be alive.

Alexis N. Misko is a former occupational therapist living with Long COVID since October 2020. Her writing has appeared in *Into the Void, The First Line, The Ides of March, Broad!, The Lascaux Review, Wax Poetry and Art,* and more.

Corie Mogenis began suffering from Long COVID in July 2020. She is a medical paralegal, an award-winning co-author of *Medical Tips From the Inside ... Things You Need to Know!,* a co-host for two local community TV shows, *Medical Tips You Need to Know* and *Wine-ing Away with Corie & Ray.* She is a metastatic thyroid cancer survivor who has written several pieces for cancer-related organizations and magazines.

Tim Murphy (he/him) is a disabled, bisexual civil rights lawyer and poet from Portland, Oregon. He has Long Covid, ME, POTS, and PTSD. Tim writes to cope, create, and to locate his voice amid the fog.

Haley Nelson is 19 years old. She was athletic, academic, and animated before Long COVID, ME/CFS, POTS, and small fiber neuropathy uprooted her life. She wants to share her story so no other woman is made to believe her symptoms are all in her head.

May Patiño had COVID-19 in December 2021. In May 2022, her Long COVID symptoms suddenly and dramatically escalated to the point that she had to go on disability. Before this, she was actively involved in her community as a university lecturer and a local and statewide Food Policy Council coordinator.

Emily Pinkerton's writing has previously appeared in the chapbooks *Natural Disasters* (2016), *Bloom* (2018) and *Adaptations* (2018), and the journals *ZYZZYVA*, *Juked*, *BlazeVOX*, and *Berkeley Poetry Review*. She is a 2023 Fellow at USF Verftet in Bergen, Norway.

Rachel Robles is a Long COVID patient advocate and contributing author to *The Long COVID Survival Guide*. As an admin for Body Politic, she helped disseminate information from leading researchers to the patient community, and is currently a member of Patient Led Research Collaborative (PLRC). Rachel is a student at the University of Bern studying artificial intelligence in medicine.

Judith Rosenbaum is CEO of the Jewish Women's Archive. An educator, historian, and writer, Judith holds a PhD in American Studies from Brown University. She teaches, lectures, and publishes widely on women, gender, and Jewish studies. She lives with her family outside of Boston.

Amy S. (she/they) was first infected with COVID in March 2020. Although disabled, they advocate for Long COVID and ME/CFS awareness and research whenever possible. Amy is a proud spouse, sister, auntie of six (soon to be a great-auntie!), cat mom, and word game enthusiast.

Christopher Soden earned his MFA in January 2005. He teaches, writes poetry and plays, and reviews theater. Two of his collections, *Terrible Grace* (with Paul Koniecki) and *Gusher*, were published in late 2022. His work appears in *Cortland Review*, *Rattle*, *Gay and Lesbian Review*, and *Texas Observer*. In 2007 his show *Queer Anarchy* was named Best Stage Performance by the *Dallas Voice*.

Jessica B. Sokol believes COVID-19 hit her in February 2020. She survived intubation on a ventilator. Her first book, *For Better And Worse*, was published in 2016. Her stories are featured in *Dorothy Parker's Ashes*, Music

Museum of New England, Forbes Library, and Valley Love Letters Project, Northampton, Massachusetts.

Morgan Stephens is a multimedia journalist and writer in Washington, D.C. She currently works for CNN's *Erin Burnett OutFront* as a production assistant, and as a freelance reporter. Her reporting on Long COVID, homelessness, the 2020 primary, and political extremism has appeared in *The Daily Beast, HuffPost, The Des Moines Register* and *The Washington Post,* respectively. She's currently writing a narrative nonfiction book and poetry collection detailing her experience with the illness and its global impact.

Nikki Stewart is a 50-year-old breast and cervical cancer educator working primarily in the African American community to combat health disparities. She lives on Long Island, New York, with her significant other. She contracted COVID-19 in December 2020.

Shell St. James is an author living in the foothills of North Carolina. Her written work has been published in several online and print publications, including *Shenandoah Literary Magazine, Hippocampus*, and *The Vanishing Point*, to name a few. Her ongoing battle with COVID-19 began in the summer of 2021.

Nina Storey is a singer, songwriter, comedy writer, and actor. She tries to use her art, voice, and public platform to bring awareness to Long COVID, using levity through music, stories, and videos, while also being an advocate for those who are disabled and immunocompromised.

Vanessa Svihla, PhD, is an associate professor at the University of New Mexico with appointments in learning sciences and engineering. Her research, funded by a National Science Foundation CAREER award, focuses on how people learn as they frame problems and how these activities relate to identity, agency, and creativity.

Dr. Stacy Wentworth is a board-certified radiation oncologist. She is a regular contributor to *Psychology Today*, addressing common concerns in cancer patients. Her prose has been featured in *Evocations*, *Women on Writing* and *DarkWinter Literary Magazine*.

Nelson White, a Long COVID survivor since October 2021, keeps the motto "Onward — and Upward" close. Leaving a career as a clinical embryologist devoted to helping build families, Nelson, a bibliophile and word devotee, began a new career as an author.

Until 2022, **John Zeising** was a career firefighter in Colorado. He first got infected with COVID-19 on the job in December 2020. A month after his infection, he returned to his job but soon found he was struggling with fatigue, heart palpitations, migraine-like headaches, and brain fog. He is now disabled and struggling with Long COVID syndrome.

About the Editors and Production Team

Kevin Barrett Kane is an award-winning book designer and type designer. He co-founded The Frontispiece in 2015 and is currently a senior book designer at University of California Press. Kevin has designed books and typography for Stanford University Press, Chronicle Books, Amazon Publishing, Dzanc Books, FG Press, John Wiley & Sons, and more. In 2020, Kevin graduated from the Type West postgraduate Type Design Program at Letterform Archive, where he co-created Wordcooker. Kevin lives in Denver but regularly spends time in the San Francisco Bay Area and Kansas City, Missouri.

Andrew David King is a doctoral student in English at UC Berkeley, where they serve as the Director of the Disabled Students Advocacy Project for the Graduate Assembly. A sub-editor of the open-access *International Journal of Disability and Social Justice*, based at the University of Leeds, their work is supported by a grant from the University of California Humanities Research Institute. Formerly Provost's Visiting Writer at the University of Iowa, they hold an MFA from the Iowa Writers' Workshop and an MA in Philosophy from Central European University.

Mary Ladd is the Long Hauler Publishing founding editor. She has written about meat clothing, withered sexuality, medical debt, and pizza champions for the *San Francisco Chronicle*, *Playboy*, *Health*, *Wildfire Magazine*, and the best-selling *642 Things to Write About* and *Lit Starts* books. Mary collaborated with Anthony Bourdain and later created *The Wig Diaries: An Irreverent Cancer Book* with illustrator Don Asmussen. She is We Wai Kai First

Nation, belongs to the Writers Grotto, and first experienced Long COVID symptoms in early 2022.

Courtney Essary Messenbaugh loves to help individuals and organizations tell their stories, connect with their audiences, and solve complex problems. She resides in Colorado and delights in the blanket of neon blue sky there. She's got three wildling teenagers, two scruffy dogs, and one husband.

Regan McMahon is a veteran journalist, feature writer, editor, book critic, and book editor who worked at the *San Francisco Chronicle* for more than 20 years, then as the book editor at Common Sense Media for almost 12 years. She is the copy editor of *ZYZZYVA*, the San Francisco literary journal, and is also a published author whose nonfiction book *Revolution in the Bleachers* (Gotham/Penguin) was named a *San Francisco Chronicle* notable book in 2007. She now edits fiction and nonfiction. Recent books she edited include Joseph Di Prisco's novel *The Good Family Fitzgerald* and Mary Ladd's cancer memoir, *The Wig Diaries*.

Tamara Palmer's career as a professional DJ—as well as a freelance writer and editor for tech, music, travel, and food publications—has been enjoyable for 30 years. She self-publishes *California Eating*, a website and small-batch print zine, and is also a cookbook ghostwriter, recipe developer, and author of a music book called *Country Fried Soul: Adventures in Dirty South Hip-Hop* (Backbeat Books, 2005).

With a background in law and neuroscience, **Meagan Roderique** brings years of experience in research, education, and international journalism. She has edited fiction, nonfiction, technical works, and for media. Currently, she serves as program manager of a health care nonprofit, where she draws inspiration from her own experiences as a chronic-illness patient.

Sydney Seymour is a Bahamian (born, bred, gon' dead) is an early career dramaturg and curator with a degree in theater and classics. She performed a one-woman comedy show, *What Happens When You Have a Stroke at 23,* about her "not-so-great" COVID-19 infection. Sydney works in New York City at *UG2MSG* (Ur Going 2 Make Something Great) magazine.

Lydia Sviatoslavsky is a New York City-based writer, editor, and publicist. She has covered arts and culture for SFGate, *Spike Art Magazine*, and the Bay City News Foundation, among others. She is an associate editor and publicist at Hyperidean Press.

Ann E. Wallace is the Poet Laureate of Jersey City, New Jersey, and an English professor at New Jersey City University. She has been writing and speaking about her family's experience with COVID-19 since March 2020 and is an editor for *The Long COVID Reader*. Ann has appeared on *Good Morning America*, NPR, CBS, and other media, and her work is featured in Huffington Post, USA Today, *Wordgathering*, *Gyroscope Review*, and many other journals. She is the author of the poetry collection *Counting by Sevens* and recently completed a new poetry manuscript chronicling her Long COVID experience.

With an uneasy nostalgia, **Michael Zipkin** remembers pasting up magazine pages onto boards armed with galleys of type, X-ACTO knives, a hot wax machine, and other analog tools of the trade. Since then, he's worked as a designer at KPIX television, built pages for the *San Francisco Chronicle*, made myriad books, magazines, and other publications, and gently guided readers with the architecture of typography. These days, most of his creative juice spills onto Bay Area dance floors, where he facilitates movement with words and music.

Acknowledgments

It's important to recognize the history of people advocating and caring for the millions who live with disabling conditions. Such help through the years brings vital resources and comfort.

The Dream Team

I'm lucky that superstar Lydia Sviatoslavsky showed immediate willingness and interest in helping bring this book to life. Since cloning Lydia remains impossible, I was elated when Courtney Essary Messenbaugh joined our wee team. Courtney is a superstar in her own right and I immensely trust and appreciate this smart and hardworking duo.

A special shoutout to Andy King for their amazing prowess with poetry, editing, and design.

When the editing goddess Regan McMahon said yes to this project, it brought many sighs of relief. Ditto for designers Kevin Barrett Kane (book cover), and Michael Zipkin (book interior) .

My respect and admiration for all things Evan Karp continues to grow after witnessing him create such a beautiful Kickstarter video!

Thank you to our contributors for writing with such honesty and vulnerability. It is an honor to read and share your stories, essays, and poems. And to our editors, each of you were critical in winnowing and finalizing the manuscript.

Community

I was excited to offer myself up as a test subject for UC San Francisco Long COVID researchers. Who doesn't love cash, gift cards, and lab results to selfishly sleuth one's symptoms?! Yet early on, I also found release and relief because the staff is kind, compassionate and intelligent. Each visit, call, and email allowed me participation in something way bigger. I deeply value Dr. Michael Peluso's enthusiasm for this book, which gave me the courage to go for it!

I keep going creatively because of the Writers Grotto community and especially: Vanessa Hua, Saila Karat, Jenny Bitner, Audrey Ferber, Celeste Chan, Julia Scheeres, JD Beltran, Beth Winegarner, Susan Ito, Fred Vogelstein, Christopher Cook, Kathy Seligman, Thaisa Frank, and Louise Nayer.

To Oscar and Cipriano Villalon, I love you.

Let's keep in touch

Thank you for reading!

Sign up for newsletter updates on upcoming books, press releases, awards, and other thrilling milestones. There may even be exclusive access to writing prompts, contests, and book reveals down the line. Stay tuned.

www.maryladd.com

www.ingramcontent.com/pod-product-compliance
Lightning Source LLC
Chambersburg PA
CBHW061154210726
48294CB00006B/1679